OUTLOOK ON
CANCER

OUTLOOK ON
CANCER

Edited by

Ronald W. Raven, O.B.E., T.D.

Former Member of Council, Royal College of Surgeons of England
Consulting Surgeon, Royal Marsden Hospital and Institute of Cancer Research
Consulting Surgeon, Westminster Hospital
London, England

PLENUM PRESS · NEW YORK AND LONDON

Library of Congress Cataloging in Publication Data

Main entry under title:

Outlook on cancer.

Proceedings of the seventh and eighth annual symposia of the Marie Curie
Memorial Foundation on Cancer, held at the Royal College of Surgeons of
England, London, England, May 13th, 1975 and May 11th, 1976."
    Includes index.
    1. Cancer–Congresses. I. Raven, Ronald William. II. Marie Curie Memorial
Foundation. [DNLM: 1. Neoplasma–Congresses. QZ200 094 1975-76]
RC261.A1095   616.9'94   77-8636
ISBN 0-306-31063-5

Proceedings of the Seventh and Eighth Annual Symposia of the Marie Curie
Memorial Foundation on Cancer, held at the Royal College of Surgeons
of England, London, England, May 13th, 1975 and May 11th, 1976

© 1977   Plenum Press, New York
A Division of Plenum Publishing Corporation
227 West 17th Street, New York, N.Y. 10011

Printed in the United States of America

FOREWORD

When the 1975 and 1976 symposia of The Marie Curie Memorial Foundation took place at the Royal College of Surgeons of England it was my great privilege to say a few words at the opening of each of them. It is equally a privilege to contribute these few introductory words to the Volume recording these symposia and I believe that it would not be inappropriate to recall with minor modifications some of the thoughts that occurred to me when I opened the symposium in 1976, for they do reflect the spirit of determined optimism, but without complacency, that characterized the contributions on both of these two occasions.

In common with many others I always looked forward, from year to year, to the Meetings and admired each time the spirit which was so apparent and so very much in tune with the general philosophy of a surgeon, the spirit which admits that to a doctor and all others who care for patients cancer is a grim and terrible foe but suggests that, rather than sitting down and grizzling about it, we should bestir ourselves, do our best, whatever the difficulties, and at least try to do a little better each year.

The title of the symposium in 1976 was typically stimulating,-"Towards a Solution",- not, admittedly a study of the solution itself but a title emphasising that the position was not static - that it was mobile, that we are moving forward and we do know where we are going.

Some years ago a distinguished British surgeon, visiting the United States, found in one centre what he regarded as a totally unacceptable degree of inertia in

the operating theatres where some lamentably slow operating
was explained by the excuse "this is a Halsted School"
(Halsted was a very distinguished American surgeon at the
turn of the century). "He taught his pupils to be met-
iculous and careful and was himself a slow operator.
What was good enough for Halsted is good enough for us".
Returning to this topic when he gave an address in the
evening, the British visitor said "You know, it seems to
me that in this centre you regard Halsted's footprints
in the sands of time as fox-holes to be defended to the
death - and re-excavated as they crumble - instead of
merely as evidence of the direction in which he was
travelling".

Today, at least I believe that we do know the
direction in which we are travelling and I particularly
applaud the refusal to become bogged down and static, the
refusal to respond to difficulty with apathy, the determination to maintain momentum in areas where progress
is being made.

"Towards a Solution".............

Yes - and if one cannot immediately reach this goal,
at all costs let us continue to move forward with determination - and with optimism.

SIR RODNEY SMITH

PREFACE

The annual symposium arranged by the Marie Curie
Memorial Foundation is concerned with an important
practical aspect of Cancer and is attended by a large
audience of members of the caring professions, who participate in the discussions for mutual benefit. The
material for this book is provided by two symposia and
comprises the lectures given by the invited speakers,
with the discussions that followed.

The book is divided into two parts. "Cancer and the
Nation" is the subject of part I. Whilst cancer affects
all nations in different ways, each has its own methods
for control, which are dealt with here with reference to
the United Kingdom. The annual rise in cancer mortality
and the considerable morbidity it causes stimulates us to
a greater effort to achieve control; there is no reason
for complacency, much remains to be done. A good picture
of the present position can be seen here.

"Cancer - Towards the Solution" is the encouraging
subject of part 2, for there are clear indications that
we are making steady progress towards this desirable goal.
There are good grounds for a more optimistic outlook
because of newer methods of diagnosis and the development
of combination treatment in addition to knowledge which
is coming from research - clinical, epidemiological and
laboratory. Bridges are now essential between clinical
and research work for the benefit of patients. We have
travelled far during recent decades, but an uphill
journey still lies ahead.

RONALD W. RAVEN

ACKNOWLEDGEMENTS

As Chairman of the Symposia it is a privilege to make the following acknowledgements for so much help and support.

The President and Council of the Royal College of Surgeons of England for the facilities provided for these large meetings. Miss Hazel Child, B.A. of the College administrative staff. Mr. Paul A. Sturgess and Dr. D. C. Williams of the Marie Curie Memorial Foundation administrative and research staff.

The lecturers at the meetings who have provided the material for this book.

CONTENTS

PART 1
CANCER AND THE NATION

Part 1
CANCER AND THE NATION

MORTALITY AND MORBIDITY

Sir Rodney Smith, KBE, PRCS

President of the Royal College of Surgeons of

England

To a doctor, the treatment of each patient with cancer presents a major problem, a problem in the application of technical skills, in the exercise of judgment, in humanity, perhaps above all in humanity. At national level, the problems are different, problems of applying resources, limited resources unfortunately, to the study of the origins of cancer and of organising services to make the maximum use of professional expertise.

No nationwide plans could succeed without a basic understanding of the mortality and morbidity of cancer.

MORTALITY

Cancer comes second in the world's killer diseases. It affects every single nation although the geographical distribution varies according to the site affected.   In the United Kingdom, reference to the Registrar General's Statistical Review, 1972, shows that in that year more than 100,000 people died from cancer, more than 65,000 men and 55,000 women, and these deaths had increased constantly during the preceding decade.   Of this total nearly one-third of the deaths were due to cancer of the respiratory system.   Indeed, lung cancer is a most serious menace to life to-day.   Other dangerous cancers are common in the digestive organs, especially in the stomach (12,443 deaths) and large intestine, excluding the rectum (10,359 deaths). In the rectum where early diagnosis and cure can be

3

expected, there were 5,967 deaths. I am myself
particularly interested in cancer of the pancreas, which is
also a dangerous disease with 5,246 deaths in 1972, showing
an increase of 1,135 deaths over 1962. It is difficult
to account for the fact that, whilst the death rate is
increasing for cancer in certain sites, including the lung
and pancreas, it is decreasing for cancer of the tongue,
larynx and uterus. Cancer of the breast, which causes
more than 10,000 deaths in women annually, continues to
cause us great concern, so that the new methods of early
detection, particularly by mammography and xerography, are
very important for the future.

This is but a brief discussion of cancer mortality,
but it does bring home the magnitude of the problem.
There are certainly no grounds for any complacency in
dealing with this situation.

MORBIDITY

The best chance of helping a patient with cancer
depends upon early detection and treatment. Many thousands
can be permanently cured, to enjoy lives of good quality
without deformity or disability. Surgery, radiotherapy
and chemotherapy, either alone, or in combination, have
much benefit to offer to patients even with advanced
disease. It is, however, distressing to find there are
still many patients in our country who delay coming for
treatment until little can be done to help them.

Reference to the Registrar General's Statistical
Review of England and Wales for 1965 gives details about
the type of treatment for cancer in different organs. It
is a surprise to find that in about 50 per cent of men and
women with cancer of the trachea and lung no treatment was
given because of the advanced nature of the disease; this
figure was about 55 per cent for cancer of the pancreas.
On the other hand, only 5 per cent of women with breast
cancer received no treatment. Considerable suffering is
caused by untreatable cancer which makes patients completely
dependent upon others.

Let us turn to the brighter side, for there are many
patients well and working to-day following surgical and

other treatment.   The development of reconstructive and plastic surgical techniques has considerably reduced both deformity and the degree of dysfunction.   Many major operations are done with a high degree of safety so that patients need no longer fear the immediate, or long term, effects.   Prosthetics have attained a high degree of perfection, minimising disability, even after a major amputation.   Biomedical research will result in even better prostheses, including powered limbs, resulting in much improved function, especially in the upper extremity.

Increased attention is being given to stomal care. Patients with a tracheostomy, gastrostomy, colostomy, ileostomy, have many different problems, which can be satisfactorily dealt with by trained stomal therapists in stomal clinics.   More of these clinics are needed in our hospitals.

Following mastectomy, patients require much supportive care including personal and family readjustment to this deformity   There are excellent prostheses to be fitted, which give reassurance to patients who feel disfigured. The leaflet for these patients available from the Foundation is greatly in demand, and is now available in French and German for the E.E.C.

Rehabilitation of cancer patients is of profound importance to-day in restoring them to family and employment, minimising their morbidity and generating hope.   The Foundation, in pioneering this vital work, has rendered a service of tremendous value and importance to the community.

NATIONAL CANCER NEEDS

Ronald W. Raven, OBE, O.St.J, TD

Royal Marsden Hospital and Institute of Cancer

Research, Royal Cancer Hospital

Spectacular advances have occurred during the past twenty-five years in the detection and treatment of cancer, which have been responsible for saving thousands of lives. Even the most serious cancers can now be cured, and many are preventable by sensible adjustments in everyday life. The growing habit of having a health check-up in middle and older age groups is helping the discovery of early cancer and precancerous conditions before the patient is aware of them, and herein lies the best chance for a cure. We have, therefore, sound reasons for optimism that cancer will be controlled provided we make a national effort. The outstanding need to-day is for members in the caring professions, researchers in many scientific disciplines, and the community to unite together to overcome this second killer disease. There is work for everyone to do in meeting the needs presented by this great medical challenge.

THE FIVE-POINT PROGRAMME

National cancer needs can be summarised in a 5-point programme -

1. Research into the nature, causation and cure of cancer.

2. Prevention of cancer.

3. Detection of early cancer.

4. Rehabilitation of patients with cancer.

5. Care of patients incapacitated by cancer.

To carry out this programme on a national scale there
must be co-ordination of effort.   There is a need to
organize closer collaboration between central government,
area and district boards, oncology centres and departments
in hospitals, community medicine and nursing, research
institutes and units, and the voluntary organisations.
The four oncology centres are given the opportunity to
organize the work in four regions, and oncology departments
can do the same for hospitals and hospital groups.
Already team-work in patient management is growing with
the realization that clinicians can no longer work in
isolation.   Surgeons and physicians with cancer
responsibilities require collaboration with radiotherapists,
chemotherapists, pathologists, immunologists, research
oncologists, nurses and other specialists in the caring
professions.   The team must, therefore, include family
doctors, community physicians, medical social workers,
physiotherapists, occupational and speech therapists,
prosthetists and Ministers of religion.   It is essential
to collaborate with the family doctors, community
physicians, home nurses, resettlement officers and the
voluntary organisations with responsibilities for the care
of patients following hospital treatment.

The professional associations: the British Association
of Surgical Oncology, the Association of Head and Neck
Oncologists of Great Britain, and the Section of Oncology
of the Royal Society of Medicine, are also working to
establish this closer collaboration.

1. Research

For the past fifty years a tremendous effort has been
expended on cancer research in animals, and, whilst this
may have scientific value, much has little, or no, relevance
in the control of human cancer.   The need now is to solve
cancer problems in humans with newer methodology by
identifying areas of research which will benefit patients.
Research workers must have some knowledge of human cancer,
which differs from the cancers they produce in animals.

Collaboration is required between clinicians and researchers; problems seen at the bedside, in the operating theatre and clinic should be fed back into the laboratories. Since the time of Percivall Pott in 1775, clinicians have detected important cancer clues; many of profound significance are still seen to-day. The fact that enormous carcinomas of the breast will heal with hormone treatment surely stirs the imagination and stimulates laboratory research to find the reason for such a spectacular result. Our hospitals and laboratories must be more closely linked together; clinicians and researchers must be in constant communication. Lay members of committees responsible for research budgets should seek some understanding of the enormity and difficulty of cancer research to give the maximum encouragement and support for workers in this field. The tremendous suffering and mortality caused by cancer throughout the world demands the maximum collaborative effort of clinicians, scientists and laymen to ameliorate mankind's distress.

2. Prevention

It is estimated that about 80 per cent of cancers are caused by environmental carcinogens, which means they could be prevented provided the right protective action were taken. Prevention is the big hope of the future. We must learn how to keep healthy and avoid disease, thus maintaining lives of good quality. Vigilance is necessary to-day about the number of chemicals eaten with our food, which are used increasingly in its production, preservation and preparation. Chemicals like benzpyrene and nitrosamines are strong carcinogens. Such substances may be connected with stomach cancer, and the number of drugs taken as medicines to-day cause some concern, because it may be another twenty years before their effects are seen. A good example was the medicinal use of arsenic many years ago, which caused cancer of the skin and urinary bladder; this usage has now ceased.

Children and young adults must be protected from cancer by advising pregnant women not to take hormones, or drugs, unless prescribed by the doctor, and the foetus should be protected from ionizing radiation. No pregnant

woman should smoke tobacco because of the ill-effects on
the developing child.

Genetic counselling is now given in some hospitals,
where there are genetic factors in such diseases as
xeroderma pigmentosa and familial adenosis of the colon
and rectum, where there is a high risk of cancer.

Lung Cancer and Tobacco.   This is the biggest health
challenge facing Britain to-day because of the raging
epidemic of lung cancer.   In 1972 there were 25,728 deaths
in males and 5,883 deaths in women with a total of 31,611.
The explosion in the number of deaths in women has yet to be
seen, for there must be thousands of these cancers
developing to-day.   If such numbers were dying from
smallpox or killed in traffic accidents, enquiries would
be demanded by the nation to stop such an appalling loss
of life.   The number of deaths from lung cancer inexorably
increases every year, but comparatively little effective
work is being done to stop it, and the sale of cigarettes
is actively advertised with the consequent rise in sales.
Lung cancer has been recognised as a tobacco-induced
disease for 25 years, but it is both startling and
regrettable we have been unable to make any real impact on
its prevention.   The time has come when we must agree on
vigorous voluntary action to abolish tobacco.   It will
take time, however, to condition people to this new health
outlook.   To begin with, the warnings on cigarette packets,
now largely ineffective, should say what is meant;   the
plausible propaganda and advertisements encouraging the
young to start smoking and adults to smoke more should be
banned, and replaced by advertisements telling everybody
how dangerous tobacco is to health.   A campaign should be
planned and executed by clinicians, health educators and
those responsible for community health to give the nation
the facts and warnings, making every effort to educate
young people in all schools about this disastrous habit.
I feel it is most regrettable that strenuous attempts are
now being made to perpetuate this human habit of smoking
by trying to produce at enormous expense what is described
as a "safe cigarette."   But what do the manufacturers
mean by "safe?"   Are the products of combustion ever safe?
Much experimentation with animals will doubtless be done
in future in an attempt to prove safety, but we shall need
to wait for at least 20 years to see how many people die
from lung cancer having smoked a "safe" cigarette.   (See

Editorial, Lancet, 1975).

In the reorganized National Health Service we have a
unique opportunity to develop health education for all.
New courses of training to supply the personnel for this
work are required; there is an urgent need for specialists
in health education, clinicians, epidemiologists and
nurses. Students in medicine and nursing need this
training, which should be included in the curriculum.

3. Detection

Many more facilities in hospitals throughout the country
are required to make a cancer check-up readily available for
people in middle and older age groups, and especially for
those at high cancer risk from habits, environment,
occupation, previous health and genetic factors. People
who notice an insidious departure from normal health
require a check-up More "well" women clinics are
necessary where breast and uterus examinations are made by
mammography and cytology. I want to see "well" men clinics
to detect cancer of the lung, prostate, and other organs
commonly affected. We now have newer techniques for this
work, so there is little excuse that so many patients are
first seen with incurable disease. One example is
sufficient to stress my plea. Carcinoma of the breast
can be detected by mammography or xerography when very
small and when it cannot yet be felt; if women were
diagnosed and treated at this early stage, I believe the
great majority would be cured.

The task of cancer prevention and detection on a
national scale is enormous, and it requires the combined
efforts of administrators, health educators, clinicians in
hospital and community, nurses and all in the caring
professions. Is it not completely logical to deal with
cancer by these means, rather than wait for the more
advanced stages to develop which require such elaborate
hospital treatment and after-care? I make the strongest
plea for a national plan and adequate provision for its
execution.

4. Rehabilitation

The object of all our treatment is to restore a cancer patient to a life of good quality and longevity. This is rehabilitation, which immediately strikes a note of hope to replace any despondency. Whilst hospital treatment is essential, there is much more to be done following surgery, radiotherapy and chemotherapy, alone or combined, by a team of experts. These are skilled in restoring function, correcting deformities, fitting prostheses, stomal care and improving nutrition. The restoration of the spirit is of great importance, in fact, treatment is directed to the whole patient. We must teach this philosophy of rehabilitation for cancer patients and provide all the personnel and facilities for this revitalizing work. I want to see such special units provided for our oncology departments, where specialist teams are available. I feel much concern for patients with major forms of paralysis caused by different cancers where so much can be done to restore mobility and self-dependence. One or two special cancer paralysis units are required in this country for this treatment, which I have seen to be effective in patients even with incurable disease. We are now seeing the most encouraging results from the new techniques of chemotherapy, and combined treatments.

Family and patient counselling require developing on a national scale by the spoken and written word. A chronic illness in a family creates the immediate need for information about the disease, its management and outcome. Leaflets are valuable for patients and their families, and are supplied by the Foundation on request. Special leaflets giving information for mastectomy patients, about nutrition and food, and general home care, are keenly sought.

5. Care of Incapacitated Patients

The period of incapacitation for patients with incurable disease can usually be curtailed to a few weeks, or even days, with our newer methods of chemotherapy. Many patients can enjoy an active life with their families, and perhaps at work if they so desire. Families often express the wish that incapacitated patients are nursed at home, and this can be done if adequate support is provided.

The Foundation has done much to meet these needs with its
Day and Night Domiciliary Nursing Service covering the
United Kingdom with 3,000 nurses on its register.   Through
the Welfare Department much additional help is given, and
all this work is done in collaboration with the community
physicians and the home nursing service.

More nurses and other help are bound to be required to
satisfy these growing needs, so the Foundation organized an
educational project about domiciliary cancer care for lay
people.   The Borough Council of Kingston-upon-Thames
approved the pilot scheme of instruction for eight weeks.
There were over twenty-five applicants for these lectures
and demonstrations (Stanley, 1972).   This course was a
big success, so I feel sure of their practical value to
lay people if similar courses could be arranged in different
areas.

Facilities for their care are always necessary for
these patients in hospitals and special homes.   The
Foundation has twelve homes with over 400 beds in
different parts of the United Kingdom.   There are obvious
advantages when such a home is sited near a hospital;   our
new home being built in Glasgow is in the grounds of
Stobhill Hospital.   The care of patients in this stage of
disease requires constant study;   there is much to learn
about giving chemotherapy;   pain and its relief;
controlling incontinence;   cachexia and nutritional
requirements;   and the relief of general suffering,
including distress of mind.   No patient must ever feel
that treatment has ceased and hope has been abandoned, and
it is important for patients to continue under the care of
the clinician who gave the definitive treatment, if this
can be arranged.   It is important to maintain an atmosphere
of hope in these homes by discharging some patients who are
able to go to their own homes for a while and readmit them
later   We must avoid the designation of a home for the
dying because patients and their families can be very
sensitive about this.

OTHER NATIONAL NEEDS

I make brief reference to other necessary developments.

A system of national cancer case records is required
in our hospitals where the details of patients' histories,
examination, treatment and prognosis are available for
computer analysis.   We need both working and research
records to avoid the present loss of valuable data.

The discovery that tumours secrete polypeptide enzymes
having profound general effects on the body, including
prostration, wasting of muscles and unconsciousness, has
enabled us to control their production, and correct the
electrolyte and other metabolic abnormalities they produce
to save many lives.   We are beginning to recognise certain
special polypeptide syndromes which require emergency
treatment.   This means bedside monitoring day and night to
measure these biochemical abnormalities and give immediate
treatment, otherwise patients will die.   All the necessary
equipment and staff must be provided for this life-saving
work in our hospitals.

I see the importance of closer collaboration with the
Royal Colleges, Specialist Associations and Hospitals for
graduate teaching and training in Oncology and other joint
work in future.

In the reorganized National Health Service we have the
opportunity of using new knowledge about cancer to save
more lives and relieve widespread suffering.   The
responsibility of the Government to take positive action
is heavy, but the voluntary organisations, who have already
done much pioneering work, can be relied upon to make a
worthwhile contribution in the future.   I trust this
combined, co-ordinated effort will be greatly strengthened
for the nation's good.

REFERENCES

Editorial. 1975. Lancet 1:618.

Stanley, P. M. 1972. A Marie Curie Educational Project.
     District Nursing. Oct. p.153.

DISCUSSION

Question 1.   Can Mr. Raven qualify the increased risk
of women who will die from cancer of the lung from smoking
in coming years?   Is the number of deaths likely to
approximate with that for men?

Answer.   We are greatly concerned about the smoking
habits of women, which have grown enormously during the
last twenty years.   It is considered likely that about
twenty-five years is the average time between beginning to
smoke tobacco and the development of lung cancer.   We have
not yet seen the full result of smoking in women and the
number of deaths is likely to rise steeply in coming years.

Question 2.   Has it been considered, and would it be
of any benefit for women, who have completed their family
and who are considered "high risk breast cancer patients,"
to have a medically-induced amenorrhoea to avoid continued
cyclical hormone breast changes ?

Answer.   I stress that women in the high risk group
for breast carcinoma should have a periodic careful check-up.
I do not advise "a medically-induced amenorrhoea," for we
have no evidence of its value in this disease and interfering
with nature can be harmful.

Question 3.   What is the state of knowledge with
regard to nutritional defects in cancer patients?

Answer.   Considerable attention is now being given to
nutrition and cancer.   Patients with different cancers
develop various nutritional defects which require treatment.
We are also concerned to learn more about small defects
which may lead to cancer.   The subject is far too large for
me to deal with in a short answer - it is rapidly expanding.

Question 4.   What is the greatest cancer risk the
people of this country are subjected to?

Answer.   The short answer is smoking tobacco and
lung cancer.

Question 5.   How do you visualize the future role of
voluntary cancer organisations?

Answer.   The future role of voluntary organisations
is just as important as in the past.   We must, however,
plan our work with vision and carry it out with enthusiasm
and vigour.   The cancer organisations have highlighted
areas in this field where much work was necessary.   For
instance, we have 400 beds for disabled patients with cancer,
which the Marie Curie Memorial Foundation has established
in 25 years.   We have also the Day and Night Nursing Service
with 3,000 nurses on our Register for domiciliary nursing.
Some of this work may eventually be absorbed into the
National Health Service as progress occurs.   We can then
look for new kinds and methods of work.   There is plenty
to be done.   One important aspect was highlighted this
morning by Sir Rodney Smith - the rehabilitation of the
cancer patient.   This subject requires much study and work
for the future.   The voluntary organisations have also made
a tremendous impact upon cancer research in the world.   A
great future is assured for the voluntary cancer organisations.

Question 6.   How can we advise patients regarding
treating intestinal delay in the aetiology of cancer?

Answer.   Intestinal cancer - cancer of the colon and
rectum - does vary in incidence in different nations.   It
is common in Europe and the U.S.A.   The evidence suggests
that it is dependent upon environmental factors.   There is
evidence that a fibre-depleted diet (low residue), which
results in colonic delay, may have some relation with tumours
in the colon and rectum.   Fibre-deficiency with faecal
arrest is responsible for bacterial proliferation and their
degradation of bile-salts to carcinogens is a consistent
hypothesis according to Burkitt, who has done valuable work
on this subject.

Question 7.   Do new advances in treatment methods,
and especially chemotherapy and combination treatments, hold
out better hope for cancer patients than previously?

Answer.   There is no doubt that tremendous advances
are occurring in the treatment of cancer.   Patients with
the most dangerous forms are being cured to-day.   For
example, leukaemia in some children is being cured by
chemotherapy;   lymphomas, including Hodgkin's disease, can
also be cured by combined treatments.   We are placing more
emphasis upon combination methods - surgery, radiotherapy
and chemotherapy.   All these methods are now being used

together at some stage in the management of many patients.
These advances give hope to patients who would have died
ten years ago, for some can now look forward to a cure.

Question 8.   Are we helping the patients with
extensive carcinoma by giving them cytotoxic drugs, which
may give them a few months of life but also cause them
considerable suffering and misery due to the side-effects
of these drugs?

Answer.   One cardinal rule in treating cancer patients
is not to use any treatment which is likely to make them
worse; this must be considered regarding any treatment for
each patient.   These chemicals we are using to-day can
cause side-effects and the greatest care and experience is
essential in their use.   This is a very specialised field
and these drugs are only given by experts, who understand
their action and who can measure and minimise the possible
side-effects.   I know one of the possible side-effects is
that patients lose their hair.   That can be distressing
for a patient, but that particular risk has to be balanced
against the possible benefit which that patient may receive;
so all these things have to be carefully weighed and balanced.
As a matter of fact, we always use a head tourniquet for our
patients so that the drug does not get through in such
quantities as to destroy the hair.   These and many other
precautions can be taken when these drugs are used.
Chemotherapy is of proven value for many patients and gives
us great hope in the future.   Doubtless new chemicals will
be discovered, which are specific for the particular
variety of malignant disease, without affecting normal
tissues and hence with diminished side-effects   Already
we are learning how to use present chemicals more effectively.

Question 9.   Could Mr. Raven enlarge on his idea of
"well men" clinics?   Are there any facilities being
provided for "well men" clinics?

Answer.   I have advocated the setting up of "well men"
clinics for some years for I do not see why the men should
be excluded from cancer screening in view of the intensive
work which is done on cancer screening in women.   The
incidence of cancer in men is high and I stress particular
sites as the lung, stomach, prostate and bowel, where
screening is valuable.   There is in this country yet no
"well man" clinic whereas we have a number of "well women"

clinics.   It is time we set up these clinics in our
hospitals, where men can go for a check-up, so that these
and other sites can be looked at.   Now we have newer
methods of screening, including fibre-optic endoscopes,
men should take advantage of them.

NATIONAL CANCER SCREENING

O.A.N. Husain

Consultant Pathologist, Cytology Departments

Charing Cross Hospital & St. Stephen's Hospital

The idea of screening for cancer in its pre-clinical state has existed now for many years but the arguments still rage over the efficacy of this approach, and certainly over the cost-effectiveness in the context of priorities for the National Health Service Budget.

In the short time available I can but touch on the salient features of the most important areas of cancer screening. (Table 1)

I should like to illustrate the problems that arise in screening programmes by considering two cancers - those of the cervix uteri and the breast - which have engaged the greatest attention up to date. A glance at the first chart (Table 1) which though not by any means complete, will give some idea of the range of diseases and the modes of attack on them, both screening and investigational. The tests can be divided into:

(1) the primary screening tests,

(2) the secondary or confirmatory tests, and

(3) the indirect or supporting or confirmatory tests. It is here that chemical, enzymatic or immunological tests will play an increasingly important part, possibly in the very initial screen of disease groups. As we will not have time to discuss these macromolecules synthesised by tumour cells plus their radio-immuno assay in

19

Table 1.

SCREENING FOR PRE- AND EARLY CANCER

CANCER	PRIMARY TEST	SECONDARY TEST	INDIRECT EVIDENCE
Cervix	Cervical smear, Irrig. pipettes	Colposcopy, Punch biopsy	Chromosomes, Enzyme (6PGD)
Endometrium	Vaginal or endometrial aspiration or irrigation	Curettage	Hormone Cytology
Lung	Sputum cytology, X-ray	Bronchial aspirate cytology, or biopsy, Fine needle aspirate, Lung scans	
Oral Cancer	Wash, scrape cytology	Biopsy	(Radio-immune assays
Gastric	X-ray, Wash cytology, Fibrescope: wash/brush/biopsy, Gastro-camera	Biopsy	(Carcinoembryonic antigen, α foeto-protein
Colon	Enema X-ray, Fibrescope: wash/brush/biopsy	Biopsy	(Foetal sulpho-glycoprotein

Breast	Palpation Mammography (Xerography) Thermography	Fine needle aspiration Biopsy	Hormones
Prostate	Palpation Massage: fine needle aspirate	Biopsy	Acid phosphatase
Skin	Scrape cytology		
Urinary Tract Cancer	Urine cytology Soluble Swab	Ureteric cytology	
Chorionic Cancer			Radio-immune assay for chorionic gonadotrcphin
Familial Nephroblastoma			Foetal nephroblastic antigen

this short account, I will refer you to one or
two recent reviews in the bibliography of this
account. (14) (26)

SCREENING FOR CANCER OF THE CERVIX

Historically, cervical cancer heads the list, as it
began when Dr. G.N. Papanicolaou discovered in 1928 that
neoplastic cells could be identified, not only from the
invasive cancers but also from the pre-invasive stages of
dysplasia and carcinoma in-situ. (39)   By 1943 Papanicolaou
and Traut had produced their treatise, devised a cheap and
simple test sample collection and developed a complex but
informative stain. (40)   The four cardinal requirements of
screening for a malignant disease (Table 2) were thus
present:

(1) the existence of a latent pre-cancer state

(2) an accessible organ to sample

(3) a simple and easy-to-perform test

(4) an economic screening procedure

The last category demands qualification in two respects

(a) an effective response from the high-risk groups

(b) a cost-effectiveness of the programme

Table 2

Cancer Screening Requirements

1. Latent pre-cancer stage

2. Accessible organ to sample

3. Simple and easy test

4. An economic screening programme

(a) effective response from
        high-risk groups

(b) cost effectiveness

There is little doubt now that dysplasia and
carcinoma in-situ are precursor states to invasive cancer,
though the proportion of these lesions that progress
towards invasion - the claims vary from 10 to 60% -
(5, 21, 23, 24) and the number of invasive cancers that are
preceded by detectable non-invasive lesions are still a
matter of considerable debate.

The latent period is variously claimed to range from
5 - 15, or even 20 or more years, and there is some
evidence to show that this preclinical stage is much
foreshortened, if not absent, with increasing age.   It is
further claimed that there is more than one disease-state
of invasive cancer (2a, 2b) and probably a variety of
channels through which the disease progresses. (41)
(Table 3)

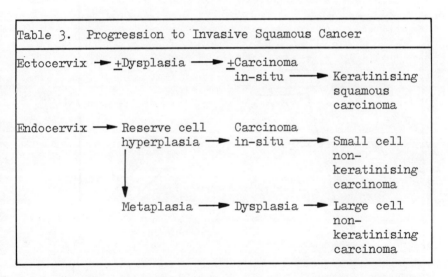

Table 3.   Progression to Invasive Squamous Cancer

Ectocervix → +Dysplasia → +Carcinoma
　　　　　　　　　　　　　in-situ → Keratinising
　　　　　　　　　　　　　　　　　　squamous
　　　　　　　　　　　　　　　　　　carcinoma

Endocervix → Reserve cell   Carcinoma
　　　　　　　hyperplasia → in-situ → Small cell
　　　　　　　　　　　　　　　　　　　non-
　　　　　　　　　　　　　　　　　　　keratinising
　　　　　　　　　　　　　　　　　　　carcinoma

　　　　　　　Metaplasia → Dysplasia → Large cell
　　　　　　　　　　　　　　　　　　　non-
　　　　　　　　　　　　　　　　　　　keratinising
　　　　　　　　　　　　　　　　　　　carcinoma

Epidemiologically, however, there is a characteristic
age-specific-prevalence-rate in those screened for the first
time, and a much reduced rate and different profile for the
incidence rate found in the re-screens of previously
negative women.   Fig. 1 shows three surveys with widely
differing rates but with an essentially similar profile.(27)

We also know that the high-risk groups relate to sexual
activity, both in amount and promiscuity, and also if

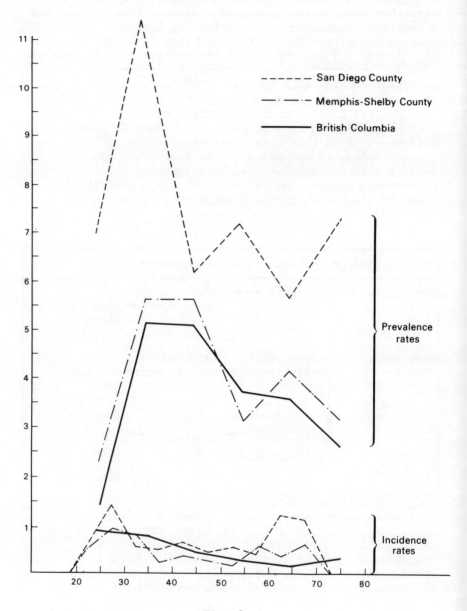

Fig. 1

intercourse commenced before 18 or 20 years of age when the epithelium appears more vulnerable to carcinogens. (5) (Table 4)

Table 4

High Risk Categories

Differential Rates Related to Single Women

Category	Rate
1. Social Class Lower v Higher	2:1 to 3:1
2. Marital State Single v Married	1:1.2 to 1:1.5
3. Multiple Partners One v more than one	1:2 to 1:3
4. Multiparity None v 1+	1:1.5 to 1:2
5. Early intercourse Less than 18 years v more	1:2, and earlier onset
6. Venereal Disease None v some	1:2 to 1:3
7. Uncircumcised) Non-sheath) contraceptive) Poor genital hygiene)	Probably increased rate

In fact, it has been found that 30% of positive smears occur in those under 35 years of age, which may indicate the changing pattern of sexual behaviour, or the use of non-barrier forms of contraception. (12) (47)   In fact, this close relationship with sexually transmitted disease is remarkable. (3)

The accessibility of the cervix and the use, firstly of the Papanicolaou aspiration pipette, then of the cervical spatula, designed by the late Ernest Ayre, which

samples the very site of development of the in-situ
carcinoma at the transformation zone, has made the test
easy and effective.   There are, however, quite serious
problems of sampling, and in some series (29) up to 50% or
more do not have cells from the endocervix, or
transformation zone, which makes the test sample potentially
unreliable.   It is wellknown that the squamo-columnar
junction, or transformation zone, is within the external os
before puberty and retracts up the canal again after the
menopause, thus making it inaccessible to the spatula.
Current opinion is tending towards requiring an endocervical
swab smear in addition to the spatula scrape so as to
collect from the canal where over 60% of the lesions exist.

As it stands, the false negative error rate in cervical
cytology appears to lie between 2 and 30% in various surveys
(29);   the cause usually being divided equally between
sampling and screener detection failure.   An aggressive
attack on quality control and training by cytologists in
this country is improving these aspects of failure.   One
cause of screener failure is fatigue from carrying out such
repetitive screening when the abnormal case may be less than
1 in 1,000.   Automation, either by fixed cell scanners or
flow cell systems, is being developed to overcome this
problem. (59)

The other problems present in all surveys is the sad
fact that those people in high risk categories are the ones
least responsive to an invitation to be screened.   As the
average response rate in this country has been around 60%,
this does not augur well for the elimination of a disease
process.   The energetic studies of social medical units
(44) (56) and cancer prevention organisations such as the
Women's National Cancer Control Campaign (60) have made
considerable inroads into the high-risk (usually the older-
aged, lower socio-economic) poor-responders groups by means
of general and personal publicity and communication, the use
of Health Visitors or District Nurses collecting at home
(38), mobile collecting clinics at the shopping centres and
homes (where the inhibitory appointment system does not
exist (60) and, finally, the use of the self-collecting
irrigation pipettes (16) (28) have all helped with different
herd groups of which our complex civilised communities are
composed.

The results of certain surveys have been of some
significance (13) and I have time only to mention two.

The largest, oldest and best-documented is that of
British Columbia.   Starting in 1949 it had screened 50% of
its population by 1964 and over 80% in the last year or so.
(4) (5)

The incidence of invasive squamous cancer is seen to
have dropped from 28.4 to 9.5 per 100,000 in 17 years
(Table 5) and similarly the incidence rate in the screened
group is 1/5th to 1/10th of that in those never screened.
(Table 6) (4)   The mortality rate (Table 7) has dropped
significantly latterly in both crude and refined rates, the
latter rate resulting from hand-checking each death
certificate to correct errors in reporting.   It is now
that a significant reduction of the mortality rate should
occur as it requires about half the population at risk to
have been screened for about half the period of the latent
pre-cancer state before any substantial reduction can be
expected in the subsequent invasive condition.

Other surveys in Aberdeen (34) and Kentucky (11)
demonstrate similar reductions and I would like to mention
our own screening programme in England and Wales in one
context.   Our national programme started in 1964 and grew
over the years to reach now well over 2½ million tests a
year.   Though designed for those over 35 years of age
every 5 years, the enthusiasm of the young and their
involvement in maternity and contraceptive clinics has
resulted in 50% of the smears being collected from those
under 35.   This means that around 80% of the young would
have been screened and only 25 to 30% of those over 35.
Now looking at the mortality rates (Table 8) you will see
that the only age group that appears to have shown a drop in
mortality is the 35-44 age group - a drop of nearly 50%.
Could this be due to the attention of the cytologists?   The
cohort studies presented by Dr. Adelstein's department (1)
(25) in the census office does not fully support this
contention (Table 9) though it may be partially the cause.

The question therefore remains: "Is screening for
cervical cancer justified?"   Our only answer can be "Yes"
if there is a detectable lesion which is likely to progress
to invasion and kill in 60, 10 or even 1% of cases, and, if

Table 5

Incidence of clinical invasive squamous carcinoma of the
cervix uteri in women over 20 years of age in British
Columbia in the years 1955-73, showing population of women
in thousands and rates per 100,000 female population.

Year	Population in thousands	Clinical invasive carcinoma	
		Total cases	Incidence
1955	422.9	120	28.4
1956	436.7	119	27.2
1957	460.9	120	26.0
1958	473.0	112	23.7
1959	478.7	108	22.6
1960	486.4	96	19.7
1961	496.0	115	23.2
1962	503.0	78	15.5
1963	513.0	98	19.1
1964	526.8	86	16.3
1965	543.2	80	14.7
1966	566.5	77	13.6
1967	592.4	85	14.3
1968	615.4	80	13.0
1969	638.2	89	13.9
1970	664.4	82	12.3
1971	687.2	73	10.6
1972	713.1	66	9.2
1973	741.4	71	9.5

Correct as of September, 1974.

Table 6. Revised incidence of squamous carcinoma of the cervix in women over 20 years of age in British Columbia in screened and unscreened segments of the population.

Year	Screened			Unscreened		
	Estimated women screened to previous year (in thousands)	Clinical invasive carcinoma cases	Rate per hundred thousand	Estimated women unscreened to previous year (in thousands)	Clinical invasive carcinoma cases	Rate per hundred thousand
1961	120.9	5	4.14	375.1	110	29.33
1962	164.2	7	4.26	338.8	71	20.96
1963	214.9	10	4.65	298.4	88	29.52
1964	260.0	12	4.6	266.8	74	27.8
1965	300.7	13	4.3	242.5	67	27.7
1966	342.7	17	4.9	223.8	60	26.8
1967	383.8	22	5.7	208.6	63	30.2
1968	423.0	20	4.7	192.4	60	31.2
1969	463.0	17	3.7	175.2	72	41.1
1970	507.8	27	5.3	156.6	55	35.1
1971	553.3	28	5.1	133.9	45	33.6
1972	593.4	27	4.5	119.7	39	32.6
1973	632.4	22	3.5	109.0	49	44.9

Correct as of October, 1974

Table 7

Crude and refined mortality rates for squamous carcinoma of the cervix in the province of British Columbia.

Year	Population in thousands over age 20	Crude*		Refined	
		No. of deaths	Rate 1/100,000	No. of deaths	Rate 1/100,000
1958	473.0	65	13.5	54	11.4
1959	478.8	65	13.6	51	10.6
1960	486.4	50	10.3	48	9.9
1961	496.0	66	13.3	51	10.3
1962	503.0	81	16.1	65	12.9
1963	513.0	60	11.7	57	11.0
1964	526.8	65	12.3	56	10.6
1965	543.2	56	10.3	42	7.7
1966	566.5	66	11.7	44	7.8
1967	592.4	52	8.8	38	6.4
1968	615.4	66	10.7	54	8.8
1969	638.2	66	10.3	45	7.1
1970	664.4	57	8.6	46	6.9
1971	687.2	69	10.0	55	8.0
1972	713.1	61	8.5	43	6.0
1973	741.4	53	7.1	42	5.6

Correct as of September, 1974.

Table 8

Deaths from Cancer of the Cervix Uteri

Year	Age Group (years)						
	0-24	25-34	35-44	45-54	55-64	65 & over	All ages
1963	1	31	316	561	570	986	2,465
1964	3	32	337	627	561	1,017	2,577
1965	3	33	330	596	604	887	2,453
1966	2	27	280	535	599	1,021	2,464
1967	3	32	241	628	574	971	2,449
1968	3	32	226	630	618	925	2,434
1969	6	32	205	564	607	1,003	2,417
1970	5	34	170	566	625	1,003	2,343
1971	2	41	184	580	594	914	2,315
1972	4	46	164	510	604	890	2,218
1973	7	39	137	542	605	919	2,249

Based on Table 17 of the Registrar-General's
Statistical Review of England and Wales, Part 1

left until it clinically presents, would kill over 50%.
It is obvious that attempts should be made to eradicate the
lesion when the prognosis is 100%.

One then comes to the realities, priorities and cost-
effectiveness. A table (Table 10) will show the wide
range of costs incurred to find one positive depending on
the age and frequency of the screen. Even this £250 per
test collection and examination is not the whole cost which,
with the follow-on investigation and treatment of minor or
major cases amounts to nearly £7 per woman screened. There
may be a cogent argument for having a differential frequency
rate for different ages and risk groups, but time is too
short to discuss this. Suffice it to say that in Oxford a
recall frequency of 5 yearly up to 40 years, then 3 yearly

Table 9.   Cohort mortality from carcinoma of cervix uteri, England and Wales.

Central date of birth	Death-rate (per million) in women aged:									
	25–29	30–34	35–39	40–44	45–49	50–54	55–59	60–64	65–69	70–74
1881										314
1886									305	313
1891								285	284	273
1896							255	246	231	247
1901						203	197	221	217	209
1906					136	181	178	193	193	
1911				93	154	187	201	201		
1915			58	119	179	204	201			
1921		30	74	134	176	207				
1926	10	37	67	106	145					
1931	9	18	44	76						
1936	5	15	38							
1941	7	19								
1946	9									

Hill, G.B. and Adelstein, A.M.   The Lancet, 2: 605, 1967.

Table 10

COST OF FINDING A 'POSITIVE'

Cost of laboratory examination	=	50p.
Cost of collection of sample	=	25p.
Hospital clinic or cytopipette	=	25p.
General practitioner (over 35 yrs once in 5 years)	=	75p.
Area Health Authority clinic	=	£2.00

TYPE OF COLLECTION	1st SCREEN 35-45 yrs 2/100	1st SCREEN 20-60 yrs 5/1,000	SUBSEQUENT YEARLY SCREENS 20-60 yrs 5/10,000
Hospital or cytopipette	£37.50	£150.00	£1,500.00
General practitioner	£62.50	£250.00	£2,500.00
Area Health clinic	£125.00	£500.00	£5,000.00

until 50 years, after which a yearly recall gave figures of suspicious or positive smears at the rate of 2.5, 3.3 and 1.8 per 1,000 women screened respectively. (52)

The cost benefit of cervical screening is unknown. The Americans have quoted that for every dollar spent, 9 dollars are saved, but this may just reflect the excessive cost of American medicine. Thorn and her co-workers (55) have quoted the cost of treating an invasive case as being double that of a cone biopsy, but this is almost certainly under-estimating the total financial consequence of the graver lesion resulting in death in over 50% of cases. Suffice it to say that screening for this lesion is justified mainly on medical, humanitarian and (now) ethical grounds, but only in a strictly controlled fashion, eliminating the wasteful tests, especially the repetitive

ones on the young, and improving the quality of sample and
accuracy of scanning.

BREAST CANCER SCREENING

At present this is the most topical and debated of the
cancer screening procedures owing to the success of the
Survey of the Health Insurance Plan (H.I.P.) of Greater New
York, (49) (53)   Here, 31,000 randomly selected women - 40
to 65 years of age in each of a test and control series -
have been studied since 1962.   This programme has shown a
1/3rd improvement in the 5 year mortality rate of the test
group over the control group. (Table 11)   The improvement
is seen to be largely in the over 50's and especially so in
the 50-59 age group.

Table 11

Deaths from breast cancer 5 years after
first invitation to be screened

(from Shapiro et al., 7th Nat. Ca.
Conf. Proc., 1973)

Age at death	Study Group n=31,000	Control Group n=31,000
40-49	13	12
50-59	16	34
60-69	11	17
Total	40*	63

*$p < 0.05$

We have similar, though smaller, programmes developing
in this country - West London and Manchester.   The West
London and New York studies are equatable in many respects
and I am indebted to Dr. Jocelyn Chamberlain for some
combined charts given in her paper to the Royal Society of
Medicine last year. (10)

In the New York series women in the study group were offered a screening examination and 3 additional examinations at annual intervals.   Women in the control group followed their usual practice of receiving medical care.   Each woman in the test group was submitted to:

(1) an interview to obtain demographic data

(2) an examination by a surgeon

(3) a cephalocaudad and lateral X-ray of each breast using a low K.V. X-ray with long and variable target film distance and close coning, on a fine grain film (M type). Radiologist and clinician compared notes regularly, though neither knew the report of the other before pronouncing on a patient.

Table 12

Percentage of 31,000 Women who responded to successive invitations for Screening.

(Shapiro et al., 7th Nat. Ca. Conf. Proc. 1973)

	Accepted	Did not accept
Initial screen	65	35
1st annual rescreen	52	13
2nd annual rescreen	48	4
3rd annual rescreen	45	3

The population response in the case of the New York series (Table 12) is a little disappointing in the first instance at 65% (for an insurance group), but the responders hold up relatively well in subsequent attendance.   Though this group is not representative of the population as a whole, it is likely there would be just over 50% response in the relevant age group.   As opposed to cervical cancer, the high-risk groups are more likely to be the ones responding.

The yield of cancer detected initially compared with
recall and expected rates are shown in Table 13.   The
excessively high initial find in the West London study can
be only partially explained by the inclusion of 200 women
invited to take part because of a positive family history,
and is being investigated further.

Table 13

Yield of Breast Cancer detected at Screening
compared with expected annual incidence

	Rate per 1,000 women	
	New York study n = 20,000	West London study n = 1,200
Detected at initial screening (Prevalence)	2.72	11.89
Detected at each annual re-examination (Annual incidence)	1.51	3.42 (provisional)
Expected annual incidence in absence of a screening programme	1.86	1.55

The success of clinical examination and/or mammography
to detect is seen in Table 14 to compare the two studies.
In New York 33% of cancers would have been missed if
mammography had not been used, and 45% missed if there had
been no clinical examination.   Only 22% were detected by
both methods.   Perhaps reflecting more current mammography
techniques in the West London series, 38% were detected by
mammography alone, 19% by clinical examination and 43% by
both methods.   The next column of the table depicts an
earlier stage of the disease by the absence of lymph node
spread, which presents the clinical method as a more
sensitive measure in New York and mammography in London,
though this is a small series to date.

Table 14

Contribution of clinical examination and mammography
to detection of early cancers

Method of detection	Number of cancers detected				Number with no histological evidence of node involvement	
	New York No.	(%)	West London No.	(%)	New York	West London
Mammography alone	44	(33)	8	(38)	34	8
Clinical alone	59	(45)	4	(19)	45	3
Both methods	29	(22)	9	(43)	14	5
Total	132	(100)	21	(100)	93	16

The false negative rate, or missed cancers, can never
be distinguished from those newly arising lesions found at
the next screen as is possible with cervical cancer.   In
New York 47 cancers were found within 1 year of a negative
screening test which represents 25% of the cancers occurring
in that group of women in that year.   West London are
screening at 6 monthly intervals to try to measure the
optimum interval between successive screenings.   So far 1
cancer has been detected 4 months after a negative check,
and 2 at the 6-monthly check.   Also in West London the
variation between different observers in both clinical
examination and radiographical interpretation is monitored.
The clinicians agreed in 54% of cases (7/13) and the
radiologists in 70% (12/17).

The other significant problem is the false positive
rate when cancer is not found on biopsy.   This may not be
wasteful as the benign disease found may need investigation
and treatment.   It does, however, come on the debit side
of the service.   In the New York study less than 1%
resulted in a biopsy for benign disease which is an
acceptable level, but in West London this is 7%, which
gives rise for concern.

The matter of the radiation dose is also important, as in New York the dose was around 8 rads per test, and though this is now markedly reduced by the newer techniques to about a tenth of that dose, it is obvious that such an application too frequently might produce a dangerous accumulation of radiation exposure if women under 40 years were introduced into the programme and a test frequency of less than 1 year was practised.

Table 15

Breast Cancer Screening
Manchester Survey

1,873 women tested in 2 group practices = 54% response
Response by decade: 6th(60%), 7th(57%), 8th(35%), 9th(22%)

	% Accuracy of Pick-up			
	Surgeons	Nurses	Radiol.	Radiogr.
379 patients referred with "lump"	81	74	69	70
71 patients with histol. proven ca.	80	65	60	60

Combined Accuracy

Surgeon + Radiologist = 89% (missed one case)
Nurse + Radiographer = 79% (missed no case)

Sellwood, R.A., 1975 Proc. Roy. Soc. Med.

The cost is also a factor in applying the preventative measures, and in West London this amounts to about £5 per examination apart from the consequential costs of biopsy of all cases, benign and malignant, and the economic cost to the woman herself.   Here the introduction of specially trained medical ancillaries, both nurses for the clinical examination and radiographers to read the mammograms or xerographs, will help to reduce the cost and some success in this field has been demonstrated in the Manchester Survey (46) (Table 15)   Here, all women over 50, in two large group practices were invited by up to 2 letters to attend

for a screening examination.   1,873 women, or 54%
responded, and this response varied by age: 60% in the 6th
decade, 57% in the 7th, 35% in the 8th and 22% in the 9th
decade.   The programme specifically set out to evaluate
the use of ancillary staff in both the clinical and
radiological tests and a team of nurses and radiographers
were specially trained to carry out the clinical examination
and read the X-rays respectively.

Using the 379 patients referred for biopsy and histology,
the accuracy of the surgeons was 81% compared wtih nurses at
74%, and the radiologists' 69% to the radiographers' 70%.

Of the 71 patients with histologically proven cancer,
the surgeon diagnosed 80% compared with the nurses' 65%, and
both the radiologist and radiographers achieved 60%.

In these patients the accuracy of the surgeon and
radiologist combined was 89%, and the nurses and radiographers
combined was 79%.

If the essential is not to miss the cancer, then the
non-medical team missed none of the 71 cases and the doctors
missed one.

A further investigation into the excretion of
androsterone and aetiocholanolone (or more conveniently 11
deoxy 17 oxosteroids) has shown them to be subnormal
compared with the 17 hydroxycorticosteroids in women who
subsequently develop breast cancer.   The abnormality is
found between 30 and 55 years and up to 9 years before
diagnosis (7) and is made more significant if associated
with the birth of the first-born child after the 25th year.
(51)   This negative discriminant of the reduced hormonal
excretion, which occurs in siblings, has been discussed in
a recent leader in the British Medical Journal 9:107, 1975.

A study of the reluctant participant in a breast
screening programme is being made by various authorities,
(18, 22) so as to improve the response rate and thus the
cost-effectiveness of such programmes.   An analysis of the
high-risk groups has been summarised from the work of Shapiro
and colleagues. (48, 49) (Table 16)   Though these factors
exist the increase in rates is not high and probably does
not affect a screening policy in view of the fact that only
50% to 60% response occurs to a screening programme.

Table 16.   Comparison of Relative Risks for Breast Cancer
Selected Characteristics

Variable	High-Risk Group	Versus	Total	White (Never married)
Marital status	Never married	Married	2.3	
Number of pregnancies	One or two	3 or more	2.0	2.5
Age at menarche	Under 12 years	15 or more	1.7	3.4
Aggregate years of menstrual activity	30 years or more	Under 30	1.4	1.6
Breast conditions (principally lumps)	1 or more	None	3.1	2.4
Familial history (sisters)	1 or more with breast carcinoma	None	1.9	1.9

Shapiro et al.   Am. J. Publ. Hlth. 58: 820, 1968.

Finally, Professor Knox of Birmingham has developed a simulated study of breast cancer screening programmes based largely on the New York series and has concluded that mortality might be reduced by up to 1,300 deaths per year in this country from the current 11,000 mortality rate from this tumour. (32)

It thus appears that regular palpation and self-palpation is justified, that there are benefits of mammography or xerography in the over 50's, that it might be dangerous to use mammography under 40 or 45 and that thermography might help before that age, or as a test prior to mammography, thus sparing the risks with the latter.

SCREENING FOR CARCINOMA OF THE LUNG

As this cancer has the highest mortality rate in the country, and this is still rising, it should be seriously considered for a screening programme. Simple 6-monthly X-rays have not proved effective in significantly reducing the mortality rate. (6) Cytologically, it is now well-known that in-situ cancer cells may appear for some years before a radiological shadow occurs. (8) Both Nasiell in Stockholm (36, 37) and Woolner at the Mayo Clinic (57) are conducting screening programmes on smokers consuming 20 or more cigarettes a day and observing the severe metaplasia and cellular atypia that occur in the sputum in advance of carcinoma in-situ. It is possible that the finding of these substantial early changes may provide the warning to cease smoking as there is evidence that a reversal of epithelial changes and improved prognosis can result.

In the Stockholm survey of 1,800 asymptomatic cigarette smokers, 6 early and clinically occult cancers have been diagnosed in a 2 to 9 year follow-up, while in the Mayo Clinic survey of over 6,000 candidates, 43 unsuspected cancers were found (a prevalence rate of 0.8%) and 13 new cancers were discovered during re-screening of the study group, i.e., 5 per 1,000 man years' surveillance. Cytology is more successful in detecting centrally-arising tumours, while X-ray is expectedly better with peripheral lesions. The use of multiple sputum samples is necessary to achieve an 80% plus reliability in skilled hands. (61)

It is considered by those workers that 5 year survival rates could be improved to more than 40%. Saccomano and his colleagues (43) have been screening the sputum of uranium miners and smokers since 1957 and all three of these surveys have been detecting and following cases of carcinoma in-situ as well as diagnosing invasive disease. They propose annual screening for such at-risk groups.

This approach has its problems, not the least of which is the problem of finding the source of the in-situ cancer cells which may subject the patient to further techniques and possible excessive X-ray exposure. Sequential bronchial washing or brushing and the use of lung scans with radio-albumins are being explored for this purpose. The enormous load of specimen microscopy would be daunting, but both improved cell dispersal and/or suspect cell concentration methods and automation of the microscopy would help to solve these problems. (59)

We await the results of these surveys and the cost-effective analysis.

SCREENING FOR URINARY TRACT CANCERS

It has been known for many years that those working in the dye-stuffs and rubber hardening industries utilising the aromatic amines (the most potent of which is B Naphthylamine) were likely to develop urothelial cancers some time in the next 15 to 30 years. (9) Periodic screening of these workers is now a national programme for this proscribed disease. In addition, it has been shown that simple fresh whole-output specimens provide an effective way of detecting urothelial cancers in those with symptoms such as haematuria. As samples are easy to collect, and automation using flow cell systems (35, 59) would be a convenient technique for these examinations, a programme of screening of high-risk groups would be appropriate in the future.

An interesting involvement of cytology is the screening and follow-up of patients who have had a previous tumour excised or fulgurated. Instead of the distress and cost of cytoscopy, cytology is presenting a simple alternative and has a better detection rate in the more undifferentiated

tumours, though sometimes ambiguous in the well-differentiated.
A substantial trial of this nature is being performed at the
Mayo Clinic at the present time at the rate of nearly 8,000
tests per year. (20)

SCREENING FOR GASTROINTESTINAL CANCER

Time does not allow comment on any but the gastric
cancer problem though the colon is becoming of significance
with the improved fibrescope and developing, though not yet
specific, radio-immune assays for carcino-embryonic antigens
and other macromolecules.

With gastric cancer the Japanese experience is the most
valuable and instructive, as they possess about 10 times the
incidence of the disease than this country.   Two approaches
exist:

(1)   that of a simple lavage via a gastric tube
      with or without mucolytic enzymes, and

(2)   the more elaborate instrumentation using
      a gastro-fibrescope.

A number of workers have achieved high accuracy with the
simple lavage method with over 90% detection rate and a very
low false positive rate (33, 45) including something like
5 to 10% of surface cancers with their much improved
prognosis.

The use of the new fibrescopes has been developed in
Japan and elsewhere in concert with the newer double
contrast X-ray techniques which in expert hands, provides
an extremely sensitive primary screen. (19, 30, 50, 58)
Fig. 2 shows the schedule followed by the Centre for Adult
Diseases in Osaka, Japan, resulting in 15,000 X-rays,
3,600 gastric camera pictures and 1,500 gastro-fibrescopes.
The cost is somewhat prohibitive even at their rate with
the price of the X-ray of Y5,000 (£7), or the gastro-camera
Y 3.500 (£5), and the gastro-fibroscopy with cytology and
histology of Y 19,000 (£27).   (Fig. 3)   Takahashi (54)
has a similar schedule, but claims a much reduced cost
amounting to £2.67 to £4.17 per case, and also depicts the
number of tests carried out in the sequence.

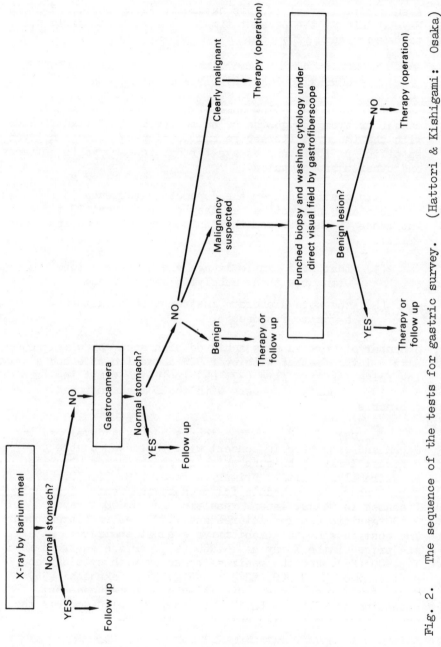

Fig. 2. The sequence of the tests for gastric survey. (Hattori & Kishigami: Osaka)

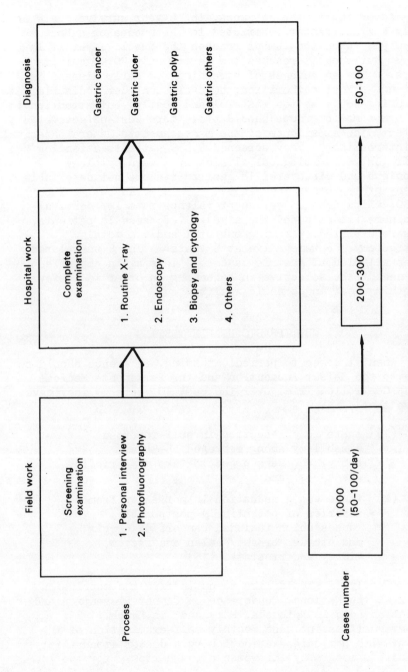

Fig. 3. Example of gastric mass survey procedure.

According to the Japanese, the 5 year survival rate of early surface cancer restricted to the mucosa or submucosa is 90.9%; when the tumour reaches the muscle layer it is 76.9%, but once it reaches the serosa only 20.9% survive 5 years. The advantages of screening for early disease is obvious. Most authorities, however, consider indiscriminate screening would be too wasteful and costly, but attention to the symptomatic groups should prove more cost-effective. In fact, the experience of the Massachusetts General Hospital is interesting. They screened 2,459 patients attending their gastroenterological clinics by a wash cytology technique and discovered 18 gastric cancers not detectable by any of the other techniques. This works out to 7 per 1,000, which equates to the prevalence rate for cervical carcinoma (in-situ and invasive). Of these 18 patients, 13 were explored, 9 having subtotal and 1 a total gastrectomy; 6 were alive at 5 years. The 5 unexplored cases all died of gastric cancer. This again emphasises the need to be selective in screening in order to achieve something near an economic reality.

MULTIPHASIC HEALTH TESTING

When it comes to periodic testing, reference should be made to the Kaiser Foundation and the Permanente Medical Group Controlled Trial over the past 10 years. They have shown that:

(1)   there is a reduction in self-reported disability among men aged 45-54 at entry, who were urged to take up periodic check-ups, and

(2)   there was a reduction in mortality from a series of potentially postponable causes which included cancers of cervix and uterus, breast, colon and rectum, kidney and prostate. (15)

Finally, I should like to quote from the conclusion given at the National Conference on Cancer Prevention and Detection held in Bethesda, Maryland, in March, 1973. Recommendations included monthly self-examination of the breast with periodic examination by a doctor or auxiliary; periodic mammography for women at high risk; for the lung,

both radiological and cytological examinations once a year
for high-risk groups, with routine examination for cigarette
smokers only.   For the cervical cases periodic cervical
smears, and for the colon, periodic examination for faecal
blood loss and proctoscopy for people over 40 years of age,
with radiographic investigation for all at high risk. (42)
In short, we are entering upon an era of positive health
where screening for early or pre-disease is merely one
aspect.   This will be successful only if and when
intelligent and discriminate use of cheap, but effective,
screening procedures, the selection of high-risk groups and
control of population response are undertaken.

REFERENCES

1. Adelstein, A.M.   Personal communication, 1975.
2a. Ashley, D.J.B.   The biological status of carcinoma
        in-situ of the uterine cervix. J. Obs. & Gynae.
        Brit. Cwlth. Vol. 73, No. 3, June, 1966 pp.372-381
2b. Ashley, D.J.B.   Evidence for the existence of two
        forms of cervical carcinoma. J. Obs. & Gynae.
        Brit. Cwlth. Vol. 73, No. 3, June, 1966 pp.382-389
3. Beral, V.   Cancer of the cervix; a sexually transmitted
        infection? Lancet 1:1037-1040, 1974.
4. Boyes, D.A.   Personal communication, 1975.
5. Boyes, D.A., Worth, A.J., Fidler, H.K.   The result of
        4,389 cases of pre-clinical cervical squamous
        carcinoma. J. Obs. & Gynae. Brit. Cwlth. 77:769-
        780, Sept. Issue, 1970.
6. Brett, G.Z.   The value of lung cancer detection by
        6-monthly chest radiographs. Thorax 23:414, 1968.
7. Bulbrook, R.D., Hayward, J.L. and Spicer, C.C.
        Relation between urinary androgen and corticoid
        excretion and subsequent breast cancer.
        Lancet II:395-398, 1971.
8. Canti, G.   In symposium on carcinoma of the bronchus.
        King Edward VII Hospital, Midhurst, 1966.
        "Some aspects of carcinoma of the bronchus."
9. Case, R.A.M.   Tumour of the urinary tract as an
        occupational disease in several industries.
        Ann. Roy. Coll. Surg. Eng. 39:213, 1966.
10. Chamberlain, J.O.P.   Implications of a breast cancer
        screening programme for a community. Proc. Roy.
        Soc. Med. 1975.

11. Christopherson, W., Parker, J.E., Mendez, W.M. and
          Lundin, F.E.   Cervical cancer death rate
          mass cytologic screening. Cancer 26:808-811, 1970.
12. Coppleson, M.   Carcinoma of the cervix - epidemiology
          and aetiology. Brit. Journal Hospital Med.
          2:961-980, 1969.
13. Cramer, D.W.   The role of cervical cytology in the
          declining morbidity and mortality of cervical
          cancer. Cancer 34:2018-2027, 1974.
14. Currie, G.A.   Human cancer and immunology. British
          Journal Hospital Med. 8:655-692, 1972.
15. Dales, L.G., Friedman, G.D., and Collen, M.F.
          Evaluation of a periodic multiphasic health
          check-up. Methods and Information in Medicine
          13:140-146, No. 3, July, 1974.
16. Davis, H.J.   The irrigation smear - a cytologic method
          for mass population screening by mail. Amer. J.
          Obstet. & Gynec. 84:1017, 1962.
17. Davies, S.W. and Kelly, R.M.   Intraepithelial carcinoma
          of the cervix uteri in women aged under 35 years.
          B.M.J. 4:525-526, 1971.
18. Eardley, A.   Triggers to action. A study of what makes
          women seek advice for breast conditions. Int.
          Journal of Health Education 17:256-265, 1974.
19. Fakuda, T., Shida, S., Takita, T. and Sawada, Y.
          Cytologic diagnosis of early gastric cancer by the
          endoscopic method with gastrofibroscope. Acta.
          Cytol. II:456-459, 1967.
20. Farrow, G.M.   Urinary cytology screening study.
          Personal communication, 1975.
21. Fidler, H.K., Boyes, D.A. and Worth, A.J.   Cervical
          cancer detection in British Columbia. J. Obs. &
          Gynae. Brit. Cwlth. 75:392-404, 1968.
22. Fink, R., Shapiro, S. and Roester, R.   Impact of
          efforts to increase participation in repetitive
          screening for early breast cancer screening.
          Amer. J. Public Health, March, 1972.
23. Green, G.H.   The significance of cervical carcinoma
          in-situ. Amer. J. Obstet. & Gynec. 94:1009-1022,
          1966.
24. Green, G.H. and Donovan, J.W.   The natural history of
          cervical carcinoma in-situ. Journal of Obs. &
          Gynae. Brit. Cwlth. 77:1-9, 1970.
25. Hill, G.B. and Adelstein, A.M.   Cohort mortality from
          carcinoma of the cervix. Lancet II:605-606, 1967.

26. Hobb, J.R.   Laboratory monitoring and screening for
     cancer. Lancet II:1305-1307, 1974.
27. Husain, O.A.N.   The early diagnosis of cancer of the
     cervix. Office of Health Economics: Early
     Diagnosis Paper 3, 1968.
28. Husain, O.A.N.   The irrigation smear.   A comparative
     trial of vaginal irrigation pipette and spatular
     smears in the detection of cervical cancer.
     Amer. J. Obstet. & Gynec. 106:138-146, No. 1, 1970.
29. Husain, O.A.N., Butler, E.B., Evans, D.M.D.,
     Macgregor, J.E. and Yule, R.   Quality control in
     cervical cytology. J. Clin. Path. 27:935, 1974.
30. Inokuchi, K., Inutsuka, S., Furusawa, M., Soejima, K.
     and Ikeda, T.   Development of carcinoma of the
     lung as reflected in exfoliated cells. Ann.
     Surgery 164:145-151, 1966.
31. Kasugai, T.   Gastric lavage cytology under direct
     observation with the fibrescope. Gann Monograph
     on Cancer Research, II Early Gastric Cancer:
     207-222. University of Tokyo Press, Tokyo, 1971.
32. Knox, E.G.   Simulation studies of breast cancer
     screening programme. In Probe to Health, ed.
     Gordon McCachlan, Nuffield Prov. Hospital
     Publication, London, 1975.
33. Macdonald, W.C., Brandberg, L.L., Taniguchi, I.,
     Beh, J.E. and Rubin, C.E.   Exfoliative
     cytological screening for gastric cancer.
     Cancer 27:163-169, 1963.
34. Macgregor, J.E., Fraser, M.E. and Mann, E.M.F.
     Improved prognosis of cervical cancer due to
     comprehensive screening. Lancet 1:74-76, 1971.
35. Melamed, M.R., Traganos, F. and Sharpless, T. and
     Darzynkiewicz, Z.   Urinary cytology automation;
     preliminary studies with acridine orange stain and
     flow through cytofluorometry.   Paper given at 4th
     International Congress of Cytology, Miami, U.S.A.,
     1974.
36. Nasiell, M.   Early cancer of the lung.   International
     Health Conference.   Addresses and Papers 23-29,
     Royal Society of Health, London, 1968.
37. Nasiell, M.   Cytology of benign change and carcinoma
     in-situ of the lung.   Tutorial Proceedings of the
     International Academy of Cytology.   Compendium on
     Diagnostic Cytology 2:253-259, 1973.
     University of Chicago.

38. Osborn, G.R., and Leyshon, V.N.   Domiciliary testing
        of cervical smears by home nurses. Lancet 1:256-
        257, 1966.
39. Papanicolaou, G.N.   New cancer diagnosis.   Proc.
        Third Race Betterment Conference, p. 528, 1928.
40. Papanicolaou, G.N. and Traut, H.F.   Diagnosis of
        uterine cancer by the vaginal smear.   The
        Commonwealth Fund, New York, 1943.
41. Patten, S.F., Jr.   Diagnostic cytology of the uterine
        cervix in: Monographs in Clinical Cytology, 3.
        Edited by G.L. Wied, S. Karger, Basel and New
        York, 1969.
42. Proceedings of National Conference on Cancer Prevention
        and Detection.   Cancer 33 Suppl., 1974.
43. Saccomano, C., Archer, V.E., Auerback, O., Sanders, R.P.
        and Brennan, L.M.   Development of carcinoma of the
        lung as reflected in exfoliated cells.   Cancer
        33:256, 1974.
44. Sansom, C.D., Macinerney, J., Oliver, V. and Wakefield,J.
        Differential response to recall in a cervical
        screening programme. Brit. J. Prev. & Social Med.
        29, No. 1, March, 1975.
45. Schade, R.O.K.   Gastric Cytology. London, Arnold, 1960.
46. Sellwood, R.A.   Surgical aspects of breast cancer
        screening. Proc. Roy. Soc. Med., 1975.
47. Singer, A.   The changing cervix from adolescence to
        the menopause. Blairbell Memorial Lecture to RCOG,
        1970. J. Obst. & Gynae. Brit. Cwlth., 1972.
48. Shapiro, S., Strax, P., Venet, L. and Fink, R.   The
        search for risk factors in breast cancer. Am. J.
        Public Health 58:820-835, 1968.
49. Shapiro, S., Strax, P. and Venet, L.   Periodic breast
        cancer screening in reducing mortality from breast
        cancer. J.A.M.A. 215:1777-1785, No. 11, March 15
        1971.
50. Shida, S.   Biopsy smear cytology with the
        fibregastroscope for direct observation. Gann
        Monograph on Cancer Research, II, 1971. Tokyo,
        Early Gastric Cancer 207-222. University of Tokyo
        Press.
51. Spicer, C.C.   Androgens and age at first birth in
        relation to risk of breast cancer, in Host
        Environment Interactions in the Aetiology of
        Cancer in Man. Ed. R. Doll and Vodo Pija, I.
        Internat. Agency for Research on Cancer (I.A.R.C.)
        Lyon, 1973. WHO.

52. Spriggs, A.I. and Boddington, M.M.   Personal
communication, 1975.

53. Strax, P., Venet, L. and Shapiro, S.   Value of
mammography in reduction of mortality from breast
cancer in mass screening. Am. J. of Roentgenology,
Radium Therapy & Nuclear Med. 117:686-689, No. 3,
March, 1973.

54. Takahashi, K.   Outline of gastric mass survey by X-ray.
Gann Monograph on Cancer Research, II. Early
Gastric Cancer 207-222. University of Tokyo Press.
Tokyo, 1971.

55. Thorn, J.B., Macgregor, J.E., Russell, E.M. and
Swanson, K.   Costs of detecting and treating
of the uterine cervix in North East
Scotland in 1971. Lancet I:674-676, 1975.

56. Wakefield, J.   Seek wisely to prevent.   Dept. Health
& Social Security, H.M.S.O., London, 1972.

57. Woolner, L.B.   Cytology of early lung cancer.
Personal communication of Abstract of Presentations.
Mayo Lung Project, 1975.

58. Yamada, T., Matsumo, O.S., Sankawa, H. and Seino, Y.
J. Am. Med. As. 228:890, 1974.

Additional References

59. Husain, O.A.N.   Automated techniques and cervical
cytology.   British Journal of Hospital Equipment,
May, 1975, No. 1:11-18.

60. Whitfield, A.P.   Cancer prevention.   Recent
encouragement in preventive measures.   Cervical
screening programmes and voluntary support.
Paper presented to Royal Society of Health
Congress, Eastbourne, April 24-28, 1972.

61. Oswald, N.C., Hinson, K.F.W., Canti, G. and Miller, A.B.
The diagnosis of primary lung cancer with special
reference to sputum cytology. Thorax 26:623-631,
1971.

DISCUSSION

Question 1.   Is cancer screening possible for large
populations?   Would it be necessary to train para-medical
workers to assist in carrying it out?

Answer.   Well, I think there is no doubt that cancer
screening is done on vast population groups, something of
the order of 2 or 5 hundred thousands.   In British Columbia
the rate is more than half a million a year.   I do not
think there is any great difficulty in establishing large
programmes - only the problem of organisation.

The question of ancillary or lay-workers, in fact, is
almost part and parcel of the whole system.   If you look at
the American Cancer Society, the Canadian Cancer Society or
any of our cancer organisations in this country, the Women's
National Cancer Control Campaign is just one of them, over
80% of the work is done by lay workers and, in fact, often
done voluntarily.   I do not think there is a means by which
one can achieve inroads into this field without the use of
voluntary labour.   In fact, the enthusiasm and stimulus
that comes from workers is enormous.   You have seen from
the breast cancer survey of Manchester, for instance, the
use of ancillary workers, the para-medicals, who can be
trained to do as well as the medicals, in fact, sometimes
better.   They are probably infinitely more dedicated to
doing that rather specific task than a hard-pressed doctor
who is literally doing everything else.

Question 2.   In view of the thousands of men dying
annually from cancer of the prostate, can you suggest any
way by which this mortality could be lowered?

Answer.   The straight answer to that one is "No."
When the Women's National Cancer Control Campaign was first
started for cervical cancer, they complained that, if it had
been a man's cancer, there would have been legislation to
fund a programme immediately and it would not have been left
to the populace to give voluntary donations.

Having said that, I should add that there have been
considerable inroads into the early diagnosis of prostatic
cancer using the fine needle aspiration technique, again on
cases that have been shown to have a nodule by palpation.

The fine needle technique is simple, causes little distress
and can be quite accurate in proving that a nodule is
sinister or not.

Beyond that, and the use of oestrogenic hormones to
inhibit further growth, I see no improvement of the
situation.   I do not think any of the macromolecule or
immuno-assay detection systems are sufficiently geared
towards this particular cancer to achieve any success as
yet, but in the various multi-phasic health centres the
prostate comes in for one of the screening techniques,
though it is largely on a palpation system in the first
instance.

Question 3.   Regarding the fall in cervical cancer
incidence in the British Columbia study, how do you explain
the similar decrease in other parts of Canada, that did not
have the cancer screening programme?

Answer.   I think the questioner is referring to a
paper by Ahluwalia and Doll in 1968, in which they compared
the results of British Columbia with Ontario and other
parts of Canada.   The authors claimed the drop in mortality
rates was due to the natural falling incidence of the
disease.   Cohort studies should also be looked at in this
regard.

In their own paper, Drs. Ahluwalia and Doll demonstrate
that 50% of the population in all three areas had been
screened by the same date, that of 1964, and it is my
contention that, unless you screen about half the
population for a pre-malignant state for roughly half the
latent period of that condition (somewhere around 10-15
years or more) you cannot expect to see a drop in the
mortality of the disease as the result of a screening
programme.   This means that about now a drop should occur,
and, if you look at the mortality rate of the British
Columbia series, both the crude and refined rates, the
reduction seems to be fairly marked in the last two or three
years.   One cannot say more than that, that it is
demonstrating the effect of cytology on top of the natural
drop that is occurring.   With any population there is
migration in and out of the country and it is in the old
and new unscreened population that the cancers are occurring.
It is here that the less responsive, high-risk groups are

the very ones least likely to come forward to be screened,
and these are accumulating in that population.

Finally, we all recognise there is more than one form
of progression of this malignant disease, some of which may
not go through the pre-cancer state.   That is the type that
is going to be very difficult to detect unless one screens
the later age groups more frequently.

Question 4.   In view of the important potential of
mammography, is this a safe procedure from the point of
view of radiation received by the patient?

Answer.   I am not sure that I am the person best
qualified to answer this question.   The problem revolves
round the dose of X-rays, which in New York was about 8 rads
a test.   With the newer techniques it is now about 1/10th
of that using either mammography or xerography.   It is
believed that xerography is less likely to cause radiation
hazards as it has a lower dose.   Whichever technique is
employed, it is largely to do with the practice and
behaviour of how it is applied.   I think the argument has
always been that one should not start using mammography much
before the age of 40 or 50 and that the frequency should not
be greater than once a year.   The West London study is
looking into this to see if they are more likely to pick up
tumours within that space of time and they are scanning at
6-monthly intervals.   This is on an experimental basis and
is using the most refined techniques.   The question of what
else might be used should be considered, such as palpation
or self-palpation as the method by which a lot of pre-
detection can take place and is free of danger.   There may
well be a use for the technique of thermography to pre-
select those cases for mammography.   However, the increased
cost of a double machine test is going to be apparent here.
The current surveys, especially that in New York, which have
been going on long enough to prove any dangers, are looked
at with some vigilance, but there has been no evidence of a
deleterious effect.   As Dr. Roe has just said, some of the
delay periods of induction of leukaemias and some other
diseases are so long that it may be some years yet before
we get conclusive answers.

Mr. Ronald Raven: I think I must call attention to Professor Sellwood's work in Manchester. He gave a very interesting resume of his work at a meeting of the Royal College of Surgeons only two weeks ago and this was one of the questions which he set himself to answer in this survey in Manchester. Is mammography safe from the radiation point of view? The answer from Professor Sellwood's work is, it is safe.

Question 5. What effect will the diagnosis of breast cancer by mammography before it can be felt have on the prognosis?

Answer. If the results of the Strax Clinic in New York are confirmed (and they are already showing signs of being so by surveys in England) there is a very good chance of saving up to 1/6th of the women aged 50 to 60 years of age with early cancer of the breast. A similar number may be saved by the palpation technique. Of course, there is some improvement in the prognosis at other ages but there is no statistical evidence to prove this as yet.

With the constantly improving techniques of body scans one hopes for a much larger improvement in the prognosis of this disease.

INDUSTRY AND CANCER

M.D. Kipling, V.R.D.

Regional Employment Medical Adviser & Honorary
Research Fellow, Department of Social Medicine,
University of Birmingham.

"It is possible that the study of occupational cancer
has led to greater advances in our knowledge of the causation
and prevention of tumour formation than any other line of
enquiry."

Donald Hunter.

The first study of occupational cancer was the work of
Percivall Pott, Fellow of the Royal College of Surgeons, who,
200 years ago in 1775, wrote of cancer of the scrotum that
it was "peculiar to a certain sort of people." The certain
sort of people were chimney sweeps.

Percivall Pott was renowned, not only for his kindness
and compassion, but also for his abilities as a surgeon.
He has found lasting fame in his descriptions of the
conditions known as Pott's disease of the spine, Pott's
fracture and Pott's puffy tumour, but for his observations
on scrotal cancer he is recognised as the founder of an
increasingly important branch of medicine (Pott P. 1775).
His observation that a definite occupational exposure was a
cause of a definite tumour was the first to be made though
Agricola in 1556 described an occupational hazard of the
lungs unaware that the lung disease included cancer. He
found among the workers in the metal ore mines of Saxony and
Bohemia that the dust had so eaten away the lungs that there
were some women who had married at least seven husbands, all
of whom had been carried off to a premature death. These
workers were exposed to nickel, arsenic and cobalt dusts,
all of which may be carcinogenic, but it is now considered

57

that exposure to radon gas in the mines was the cause of
cancer of the lung.   An increased incidence of lung cancer
in uranium miners, fluorspar miners in Canada and haematite
miners in Cumberland is attributed also to radon gas.

Occupational cancers are comparatively few in number
but the identification and study of their incidence is of
the greatest importance in the study of cancer as a whole.
They are unique in that their cause can be identified and
removed, the degrees of risk from varying exposures may be
measured from past histories and the relationship of
aggravating or modifying factors may be studied.   A most
important aspect, however, is that starting with Pott's
observations on soot, it has been possible to isolate
chemically the active carcinogenic agents in pitch, tar and
oil, and this study has been the basis of all our chemical
research on cancer.

Pott noted that cancer of the scrotum, a rare tumour,
was peculiar to a certain sort of people, a definite
occupational group, and similar observations have led to
the identification of the majority of occupational tumours.
Experiments on animals and statistical studies have so far
been of little value in raising suspicions that a hazard
exists though, once this has occurred, large scale
epidemiological studies are essential for obtaining further
evidence.   Pott's observation was followed by that of
Sir Henry Butlin, a surgeon at St. Bartholomew's Hospital,
who, in 1892, described skin cancer in the pitch and tar
industry, and by Dr. Joseph Bell (1876) in shale oil workers
in Scotland.   Conan Doyle, one of Joseph Bell's medical
students, was sufficiently impressed with his powers of
observation to take him as his model for Sherlock Holmes.
In 1910 a young surgeon in Manchester wrote on cancer of the
scrotum in mule spinners of cotton - a serious and widespread
condition which caused, at the very least, over 500 deaths,
and led to the intensification of efforts to isolate the
carcinogens in oil, pitch and tar, resulting in the
identification of such carcinogenic polycyclic hydrocarbons
as benzo(a)pyrene (Henry S.A. 1946).   The virtual
disappearance of mule spinner's cancer, due to preventative
measures and the decline of the industry, was followed by an
increased incidence of scrotal cancer among automatic
machine setters and operatives in the Birmingham region.
These workers, together with some in other trades, such as

Table 1.   Expected and observed number of subsequent
            primary tumours in men with oil exposure.

	Expected Number	Observed Number	P
All sites	8.24	28	0.001
Larynx	0.13	2	0.05
Bronchus	2.64	11	0.001
Skin	0.77	11	0.001
Remainder	4.70	4	n.s.

Dr. A.H. Waldron.

metal rolling and hardening, were exposed to continuous
contamination with neat oils and the numbers affected rose
to a maximum of about 15 cases a year, of which 50% were
fatal.   The risk was found to occur in occupations in
which oil was used, that had not been treated by solvent
refining and the subsequent removal of the major portion of
polycyclic hydrocarbons.   A study of fatal cases suggested
that other tumours elsewhere in the body occurred in cases
with cancer of the scrotum and that these tumours were not
secondary to the original growth.   Statistical investigation
by Dr. J.A.H. Waterhouse of the Birmingham Cancer Register
showed that there was an excess of cancer of the lung and
digestive tract, and it is thought this was connected with
the frequent presence of oil mist in the atmosphere of some
engineering shops.   An excess of lung tumours had been
previously reported in mule spinners, and shown to occur in
coal-tar and pitch workers, particularly in retort house
workers in the manufacture of coal gas (Doll R. 1952).

        The observations by Drs. C.A. Sleggs and J.C. Wagner in
South Africa in 1956 revealed a hitherto completely unknown
and unsuspected carcinogenic hazard in industry.   They
noted that a number of cases of an obscure type of disease
of the pleura of the lung in one hospital, came from the

same district and showed that this disease was connected
with proximity to certain asbestos mines, and was caused by
a progressive malignant condition - a mesothelioma
(Wagner J.C., Sleggs C.A. and Marchand P. 1960). Wagner's
further work with members of the Pneumoconiosis Research
Unit at Cardiff showed that previous cases of this same
growth in Great Britain were clustered around areas where
asbestos was used, such as asbestos works and shipbuilding,
and that exposure to blue asbestos - crocidolite - was the
cause.   All crocidolite mines were not centres of an
increased incidence of mesotheliomata but only those in
which the crocidolite was of a particular physical
characteristic - a small diameter.   It has been shown that
mesothelioma may occur after as little as six weeks exposure
to crocidolite.   Unlike the cancer of the lung that was
found to occur in cases of asbestosis - in up to 60% of
cases in 1964 - there is no connection with fibrosis of the
lungs.   The incubation period may be prolonged for at least
thirty years as has been demonstrated by cases now occurring
in Nottingham (Jones J.S.P. 1974).   Approximately 30 men
and women, who worked for a short period in the war making
gas mask filters, have developed mesotheliomata, of whose
origin there is no doubt since the asbestos fibres in their
lungs can be shown to have originated from a particular
crocidolite mine - now closed - in Western Australia.
Epidemiological investigations have shown that the
development of cancer of the lung in cases of asbestosis
is largely dependent on cigarette smoking, and that in
asbestos workers there is a slight but significant excess
of laryngeal and gastro-intestinal tumours, but that these
findings do not apply to the incidence of mesotheliomata.
Mesotheliomata are rare tumours, of which at least 85% can
be attributed to asbestos exposure.   By 1968, 550 cases
from this exposure had been identified in Great Britain,
but with a long latent period for development it must be
some time until preventative measures cause the disappearance
of the disease.

        Recently another very unusual tumour - angiosarcoma of
the liver - has been shown to be caused, in some cases, by
industrial exposure to vinyl chloride.   This gas, which
was used experimentally in the United States as an
anaesthetic, is polymerised to form polyvinyl chloride, PVC,
a plastic of infinite use, of which approximately 10,000,000
tons are now made throughout the world annually.   In the

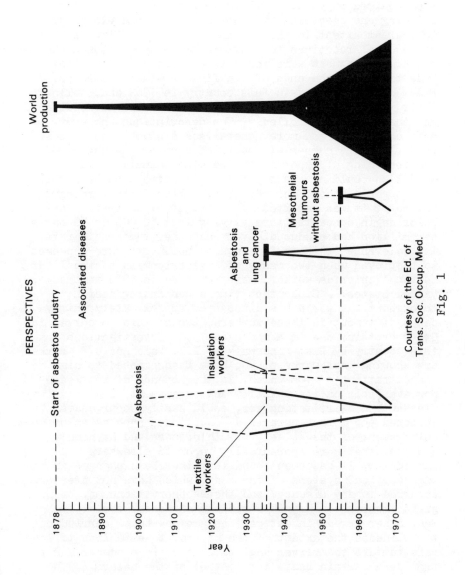

Fig. 1

manufacture, vinyl chloride monomer is converted in
autoclaves to the PVC powder which is moulded by heat into
the required objects.   PVC is used extensively in the
building and electrical trades, furniture and clothing, and
to a great extent in the car industry.   The first suspicions
of abnormal reactions to vinyl chloride were aroused when
autoclave cleaners were found to be suffering from loss of
bone tissue at the ends of the fingers - acro osteolysis.
A few cases occurred in this country in 1965 and, following
their recognition, precautionary methods were introduced
and the hazard controlled.   The descriptions, however, of
acro osteolysis and more generalised disturbances in some
factories in a number of countries resulted in the
commissioning of experimental work on animals.   The
condition could not be reproduced in animals but a possible
carcinogenic hazard was revealed.   From further research
in Italy, it was reported in 1974 that exposure to vinyl
chloride in concentrations varying from 10,000 to 50 parts
per million had produced liver and other tumours in rats.
The relevance of these findings to human exposure appeared
to be proved when two cases of angiosarcomata of the liver
in vinyl chloride workers were reported in 1974 in the
United States.   Since that time a continuing search
throughout the world has discovered approximately thirty
cases of tumour in these workers, two of which occurred in
Great Britain, one in a man aged 75.   Investigations in
this country by Drs. Anne Walker, P.T. Vale and C.S. Darke
are showing that workers, who have been exposed to high
concentrations of VCM which, in the absence of knowledge
now available on its toxicity and because it is a relatively
pleasant, non-irritating gas, could easily occur, have
suffered the more generalised conditions, such as scleroderma,
enlargement of the spleen, breathlessness and Raynaud's
disease, that were sporadically reported elsewhere.   In
particular, it has been found that there are changes in the
immunological systems of the body, which have not previously
occurred in any disease, and these observations may be of
great importance in future studies on cancer formation.
Many other urgent investigations are now being carried out
to delineate the extent of the hazard, to establish if less
rare tumours than liver angiosarcomata are produced and to
provide a certain basis for control of the hazard.   The
discovery of a carcinogenic hazard in the use of VCM, a
simple chemical substance, has led to reconsideration of
many other similar substances in industry.

Table 2. Reported cases of angiosarcoma of the liver among vinyl chloride polymerization workers.

Country	Case	Age at Diagnosis	Total Years Exposure
Canada	01	*	*
Canada	02	*	*
Canada	03	*	*
Canada	04	*	*
Czechoslovakia	01	*	*
Czechoslovakia	02	*	*
France	01	43	19
Great Britain	01	71	20
Great Britain	03	38	4
Italy	02	43	6
Norway	01	56	21
Rumania	01	*	*
Sweden	01	43	18
United States	01	49	16
United States	02	36	13
United States	03	58	28
United States	04	43	15
United States	05	52	18
United States	06	45	12
United States	07	45	18
United States	08	41	15
United States	09	43	17
United States	10	55	17
United States	11	61	23
United States	12	50	15
United States	13	53	30
United States	16	41	4
United States	17	43	19
West Germany	01	40	11
West Germany	02	38	13
West Germany	04	44	11
West Germany	05	49	11

* Data not yet available.

Another tumour that occurs as rarely in nature as
cancer of the scrotum is cancer of the nose and its appearance
in nickel refiners in South Wales in two patients, noted by
the local doctor in 1905, led to further investigations.
The eventual finding was that cancer had appeared within
thirty years of the opening of the nickel refining plant and
that there was an increase of 150-fold for nasal cancer and
a 5-fold increase for lung cancer among these workers.
Modifications and improvements in the plant and its working
removed the hazard.   At first it was considered that the
nickel carbonyl gas in the process was the carcinogen, but
the occurrence of cases of cancer in a different process in
Canada suggests that other nickel compounds are carcinogenic.
Two other examples of an increased incidence in nasal cancer
have been recently discovered in this country.   Miss E.
Hadfield, FRCS, realised that a number of cases of
adenocarcinomata of the nose were occurring in the High
Wycombe area and an investigation found that their occupation
was in the furniture industry.   It would seem that
continuous exposure to wood dust in the past was the possible
cause (Hadfield E.H. 1970).   A further study of the
geographical incidence of nasal cancer in the same region
showed another small but definite excess in the
Northamptonshire area connected with the leather industry.

An increased incidence of cancer of the lung has been
reported in workers in the chromate industry from a number
of countries.   In 1949 and again in 1956 surveys were
carried out among the small number of workers in this
country.   It was concluded that the incidence of lung
cancer was increased between 3- and 4-fold and that the
agent was an intermediate product in the production of
chrome compounds from the metal ore.   Work is continuing
on the identification of possible carcinogenic chrome
compounds in chromate production and in the use of chrome
compounds (Bidstrup P.L. and Case R.A.M. 1956).

Among the most important carcinogens in industry in
terms of numbers affected were the aromatic amine compounds.
It was recognised in Germany 80 years ago that aniline or
its derivatives were the cause of bladder tumours, and in
1918 and 1926 Dr. J.C. Bridge, the Senior Medical Inspector
of Factories, reported the occurrence of bladder tumours in
the British dyestuffs industry.   In 1948 Dr. R.A.M. Case
was asked by the Association of British Chemical

Manufacturers to carry out a full scale survey.   He found
that there had been 341 workers who had developed bladder
tumours, of whom 87% had been in contact with benzidine, or
1 or 2 naphthylamine, and also that the risk of bladder
tumour was thirty times greater in this population than in
the general population.   It was confirmed that magenta and
auramine manufacture also produced a hazard (Scott T.S.
1962).   Fortuitously in this survey, Case used as controls
some statistics from a population that contained rubber
workers, and, as a result, found there was a very definite
increase of bladder cancer in these workers due to the use
of an antioxidant that was contaminated with 2 naphthylamine.
Because of this finding, the antioxidant was withdrawn in
1949 and the exposed population afforded the facilities of
cytological testing of the urine.   Dr. H.G. Parkes, the
Medical Director of British Rubber Manufacturers Health
Research Unit, is monitoring an exposed population of 20,000.
He has records of 659 occupational bladder cancers altogether.
A Department of Employment survey showed that in a 5-year
follow-up of 40,867 subjects in the rubber and cable making
industries, there was no increased mortality from cancer of
the bladder in those employed after 1949.   There has been
exposure to bladder carcinogens in occupations other than in
the dyestuffs and rubber industries though to a much lesser
degree.   They include the manufacture of security paper,
organic pigments, rat poisons, coal gas manufacture and in
laboratories.   Benzidine was well known to medical students
and nurses as a reagent for testing for blood.   Since 1967
the use and importation of the known bladder carcinogens has
been statutorily banned and the suspected carcinogens
controlled in this country, but, with a latent period for
development of up to forty years, occupational bladder
cancer cannot be expected to disappear immediately.

Arsenic has been known to be a carcinogen when taken
over many years as a medicinal tonic, producing skin tumours
on the palms of the hands and soles of the feet, but the
only reports in this country of an occupational hazard were
of cancer of the scrotum in tin refiners in 1820 and in 1925
of 7 cases of lung cancer in an area containing a sheep dip
factory.   Recent accounts from America of cancer in two
factories have removed some of the doubts that were held on
the value of earlier findings.

To complete the list of cancers that have been caused

by occupations in Great Britain, there must be added cancer
of the skin from over-dosage of radiation in the early years
to X-ray workers, and leukaemia from the solvent benzene has
been reported.   Hazards reported other than in Great
Britain, such as lung cancer from bis-chloromethylether in
ion exchange resin workers, and of the possibility of a
carcinogenic effect in man as from the use of MBOCA,
methylene-bis-ortho-chloroaniline, in foam plastics, have
led to intensive searches for similar risks in this country
and the application of full preventative measures.

Prevention of occupational cancer hazards requires
that any suspicion that a risk exists, be substantiated by
retrospective and prospective epidemiological surveys,
processes which, because of the statistics available in
government departments and in some regional cancer registers,
this country is unique in its ability to undertake.   If a
carcinogenic hazard exists, it may be removed by statutory
prohibition, as for bladder carcinogens, or by the setting
of a threshold limit value for the substance in atmosphere,
that may not be exceeded.   The efficacy of preventative
measures may be monitored by continuing surveillance, as
has been done for those exposed to bladder carcinogens and
asbestos.   For cancer due to oil, reliance has been placed
on advice to use solvent refined oils and the very widespread
distribution of a warning leaflet to ensure recognition and
early treatment of any lesion on the scrotum.   Warning
leaflets are also available for those working with oil in
mule spinning, pitch and tar, asbestos and MBOCA.

I think it is true to say that in the control of
occupational carcinogenic hazards "the proper study of
mankind is man."   The extrapolation of data from animals
to man is still wrapped in obscurity, and measurements of
the environment may not have a clear meaning;   for example,
in exposure to polycyclic aromatic hydrocarbons from tar and
oil, the most studied of all carcinogenic agents, the authors
of an International Agency for Cancer Research Monograph
state that "no prediction as to human cancer risks may be
made from a simple knowledge of the levels of polycyclic
aromatic hydrocarbons in the environment."   Finally, in this
meeting to discuss Cancer and the Nation, it is a pleasure
to state that Great Britain is generally considered to be the
world leader in this branch of medicine - a fitting memorial
to Percivall Pott.

REFERENCES

Agricola, G.   1556.   De Re Metallica, Basel.

Bidstrup, P.L. and Case, R.A.M.   1956.   Carcinoma of the
    lung in workers in the bichromate-producing industry
    in Great Britain. Brit. J. Ind. Med. 13:260.

Doll, R.   1952.   The causes of death among gas workers
    with special references to cancer of the lung. Brit.
    J. Ind. Med. 9:180.

Hadfield, E.H.   1970.   Adenocarcinomata of the para-nasal
    sinuses. Ann. Royal College of Surgeons 46:301.

Henry, S.A.   1946.   Cancer of the scrotum in relation to
    occupation.   London.   Oxford University Press.

Hunter, D.   1955.   Diseases of occupations.   English
    Universities Press 716.

International Agency for Research on Cancer.   1973.
    IARC Monographs on the evaluation of carcinogenic
    risk of chemicals to man 3:34.

Jones, J.S.P.   1974.   Pathological and environmental
    aspects of asbestos-associated diseases. Med. Sci. and
    Law 14:152.

Pott, P.   1775.   Cancer scroti in Chirurgical Observations.
    London.   Hawes, Clarke and Collins 5:63.

Scott, T.S.   1962.   Carcinogenic and chronic toxic
    hazards of aromatic amines.   Amsterdam.   Elsevier
    Publishing Company.

Wagner, J.C., Sleggs, C.A. and Marchand, P.   1960.
    Diffuse pleural mesotheliomata and asbestos exposure
    in the North West Cape Province. Brit. J. Ind. Med.
    17:260.

DISCUSSION

Question 1.   How do the safety precautions against
cancer in industry in the United Kingdom compare with those
in other countries?

Answer.   In my opinion we are well ahead of any other
country, although obviously there may be personal bias.

Question 2.   How close is the collaboration between
doctors in industry and research oncologists so that clues
can be referred at once to the laboratory for further
investigation?

Answer. I think as far as our governmental departments are concerned, they are very close. For example, personally I am much connected with Birmingham University, Department of Cancer Research, and there are constant goings and comings between us. On a higher scale, Dr. Owen of our department takes a great part in the Medical Research Council and other activities on this subject. Works doctors, also, as soon as they suspect anything, will go straight to the expert for advice. I think the connection is extremely close because we want to find out all we can to prevent, and, as a whole, oncologists are longing to hear about anything that could have any relevance to the cause of cancer, and they are delighted if we take anything that could in any way be the cause of cancer.

Question 3. In cases of carcinoma of the lung in asbestos workers, is the carcinogen asbestos itself or a contaminant?

Answer. The precise mechanism is not know but, as regards crocidolite and mesothelioma, it seems more and more likely that it is to do with the physical characteristics. Crocidolite is composed of little fibres which are almost unique, and mesothelioma may be very strongly related to the physical conditions of the inhalation of this very, very fine fibre.

Question 4. What is the extent of monitoring the possible effects of industrial carcinogens in workers to-day?

Answer. There are two parts. Monitoring first of all is the consideration of whether substances are likely to be carcinogenic and this is, of course, greatly increasing with the increasing interest. It is very hard to forecast whether a substance will be carcinogenic. As an example, the new material that has been in use for a few years in foam plastics, called MBCOA, has been thought to be carcinogenic because it does resemble chemically-known aromatic amines that cause bladder cancer, and there are some reports of a possible haematuria in humans. As a result of this consideration, it has been advised that it either should not be used or, if used, with extreme caution. In fact, our department has issued a leaflet on it, advising how it should be used, although it is not a proven carcinogenic agent. That is one kind of monitoring.

The other monitoring, of course, is monitoring people
and this really means getting lists of those who have been
exposed to possible carcinogens and following the cancer
experience of this group.   This is a very sensitive
measure of following people up and is being done on an ever
increasing scale.

Question 5.   What screening tests, if any, are
available to screen workers exposed to vinyl chloride monomer?

Answer.   There is a code of practice, published by our
department in consultation with the TUC and CBI, on measures
taken for vinyl chloride.

Question 6.   What measures can be taken for screening?

Answer.   There are quite a number that may be taken.
For example, for the finger bone changes, some people have
X-rayed the hand at regular intervals.   For Raynaud's
disease, and thickness - scleroderma - of the skin, it is
possible to do skin temperature tests at regular intervals.
Another test is the estimation of liver function.   These
are biochemical tests and they really have not been proved
yet to be of certain value.   There are also the ultrasonic
machines for measuring the liver to estimate any increase
in size or shape, and these are possibly of value but they
are not widespread and are extremely expensive.   Blood
changes have been described in these workers abroad,
particularly thrombocytopenia, and, therefore, I think
blood tests are a reasonable regular test.   People have
described changes in lung function and in some countries
abroad they have done routine lung function tests.   There
are many vague symptoms which may or may not be connected
with exposure to fairly high doses of this vinyl chloride
monomer, and I think an important screening test is to see
everyone when they start work and to see them whenever they
have been off, to get details.   Finally, with any screening,
the important thing is to get names and get lists of everyone
who has been exposed in the manufacture of PVC and VCM.

Question 7.   Are merchant seamen working on oil or gas
tankers a high-risk group?

Answer.   I do not know of any particular risk nor would
I expect there to be one.

Question 8.   What is the risk of bladder cancer from smoking?   Please give type of cancer prognosis.

Answer.   There is an increased risk but I cannot give any exact figures.   For bladder cancers in rubber workers, the British Rubber Manufacturers Association found that 63% of a sample had a survival rate in excess of 5 years.

Question 9.   Is a uniform system of documentation kept in this country on workers in industry developing cancer?

Answer.   The provision of methods of uniform documentation are being studied at the present time.

CHANGING RISKS IN THE UNITED KINGDOM

Francis J.C. Roe

Consultant in Cancer Research

Huntingdon Research Centre, England

Two areas of change in society likely to be reflected during the years to come in changes in cancer risk merit our attention to-day. The first is closely related to the contribution of the previous speaker and concerns the growing awareness by the general public and by responsible authorities that chemicals to which people are exposed at work may increase their chances of developing cancer. The second concerns the possible risk of cancer from the use of sex hormones.

THE HEALTH AND SAFETY AT WORK ACT, 1974

In 1974, the passing of the Health and Safety at Work Act made it, for the first time, the statutory duty of "any person who manufactures or supplies any substance for use at work - (a) to ensure, so far as is reasonably practicable, that the substance is safe and without risks to health when properly used, and (b) to carry out or arrange for the carrying out of such testing and examination as may be necessary for the performance of the duty imposed on him by the preceding paragraph." This means, as I see it, that it is not now lawful for an employer to allow employees to be exposed to a substance in such a way that it might reasonably be suspected of constituting a cancer risk. Moreover, the onus is now squarely on him, where there is any doubt, to make sure that the use of a chemical in his factory does not constitute a cancer hazard. If this had been the law a century ago, and if we had had then the knowledge we have now of the mechanisms involved in cancer

71

causation and of how to test chemicals for carcinogenic
activity, we might not have seen some of the tragic examples
of occupational cancer, which Dr. Kipling described in his
paper.   It is important, however, to point out that the new
Act also prescribes statutory duties for the employee:-
"It shall be the duty of every employee at work to take
reasonable care for the health and safety of himself and of
other persons who may be affected by his acts or omissions
at work," etc.   Occupational hygienists and safety officers
are all too aware of the difficulties of persuading workers
to protect themselves from exposure to dusts, fumes and oils.
Workers complain that protective clothing is cumbersome and
restrictive, and find it difficult to believe that exposure
to an apparently bland dust or fluid, when they are aged only
20 or so, may determine whether or not they develop a cancer
when they are 50.   Moreover, in Britain some groups of
manual workers do not have a good record as far as standards
of personal hygiene are concerned.

In 1892, Henry Butlin gave a series of three lectures
on cancer of the scrotum in chimney-sweeps and others
(Butlin, 1892).   In the second of these lectures, he
discussed why foreign sweeps do not suffer from scrotal
cancer in the same way as sweeps in Britain do.   He
concluded that higher standards of personal hygiene,
especially in Germany, was an important factor.   The
following descriptions make the point clearly.   Butlin has
this to say of the life-style of English sweeps.   "I have
been informed by the daughter-in-law of a sweep that the
"old man" was very clean and had a bath all over every night
after his work.   But this, so far as I have been able to
ascertain from the men or their families, is a great
exception to the general rule.   The houses of the sweeps
and the rooms in which they live are often extremely dirty...
The dirt was so great in some of the rooms which I visited
that, in spite of the care and politeness of the people, I
found it difficult to stand without soiling my clothes with
soot-dirt."   By contrast, Butlin gives us this description
of the way a master sweep in Germany lived in the 1890's.
"In Hanover, a master sweep, Herr Fricke, was visited.   He
lived on the third floor of a tall house in a small street.
The living rooms were exceedingly clean.   The journeymen
washed after their work was over in a small room where there
were three or four wooden tubs.   They stood in the tubs and
washed with warm water, soap, and even soda, from head to
foot every day."

Table 1.   Influence of social class on cancer mortality.
Standardized mortality ratios for men and
women aged 15 - 64 from all forms of cancer.

Social Class	Men	Women
I	73	89
II	80	92
III	104	103
IV	102	100
V	139	124

from Registrar General's Decennial Supplement, 1961.

As our cities become cleaner, as those who live in
slums are provided with bathrooms and with better, warmer
houses, which offer the possibility of privacy, it is
reasonable to hope that personal hygiene standards will
rise.   As a result, the incidence, not only of various
infectious diseases, but also of some forms of cancer is
likely to fall.   It is a fact that several kinds of cancer
occur in higher incidence among men and women in social
class V than among those of social classes I or II.
(See Tables 1 - 3)

It is, then, reasonable to hope that the observance of
the 1974 Safety and Health at Work act, coupled with
improved standards of personal hygiene, generally will, in
the long run, reduce the risk of cancers due to exposure,
not only to presently known carcinogens, but also to as yet
unrecognised industrial carcinogens.   However, this hope
will only be fully realised if employees, as well as
employers, fulfil their obligations.   In any case, any
improvement can not be dramatic because many people, who at
present enjoy good health, have already had the seeds of
industrial cancer sown in them by reason of their past
exposure to carcinogens, such as asbestos, vinyl chloride,
mineral oils, etc.   Even though such people may no longer
be exposed to these agents, they are incubating cancers
caused by this past exposure.   Only when all these cancers
have manifested themselves, can we hope to see real benefits

Table 2. Influence of social class on standardized mortality ratios for cancers of specific sites in men aged 15 – 64.

Social Class	Stomach	Lung	Bladder	Large Bowel	Prostate	Brain
I	49	53	80	120	103	119
II	63	72	79	99	107	98
III	101	107	106	105	99	102
IV	104	104	104	92	96	96
V	163	148	127	109	116	112

Table 3. Influence of social class on standardized mortality ratios for cancers of specific sites in women aged 15 – 64.

Social Class	Stomach	Lung	Rectum	Breast	Uterine Cervix	Body of Uterus
I	50	83	69	111	34	103
II	76	89	81	104	64	99
III	103	102	107	104	100	103
IV	110	101	106	96	116	98
V	153	131	132	104	181	110

from Registrar General's Decennial Supplement, 1961.

from the new law.   In the meantime, however, we can and
should be doing our best to identify people who have been
exposed to known carcinogens at work, and to observe them
closely so that appropriate treatment can be instituted at
the earliest stage of the disease when it has the best
chance of success.

One other aspect of the passing of this law merits our
attention.   There are people - certainly more vociferous
than numerous - who believe sincerely that it is morally
wrong to use animals for experimental purposes, and,
therefore, decry their use for testing chemicals and other
agents to see if they cause cancer.   I am not entirely
without some sympathy for this view, and certainly accept
that it is the prerogative of society as a whole, provided
that it is adequately appraised of the issues and facts, to
decide whether animals should or should not be used for such
purposes.   Over twenty-five years experience, both of the
practice of medicine and of experimental cancer research,
leaves me personally in no doubt as to what is right and
what is wrong.   Most cancer tests on animals cause them at
most no more than intermittent and minor distress.   By
comparison, one premature death of the wage-earner of a
family can be a bitter tragedy.   I am, therefore, in no
doubt that it is right to test suspect chemicals, to which
men are liable to be exposed at work, for carcinogenicity.
As far as possible, such tests should be conducted in
purpose-bred laboratory animals and not in animals caught
in the wild, for whom captivity itself is stressful and
which, being of undeterminate age and background, are not
entirely suitable for precise scientific studies anyway.
At the present time, there simply is no other way by which
carcinogenically dangerous and carcinogenically safe
chemicals can be satisfactorily distinguished.   Hopefully,
in the future, an increased knowledge of the mechanisms
involved in cancer production will enable us to dispense
with the use of animals.   Until then it would be
inappropriate to bask in the moral luxury of regarding
animal tests as barbaric.

In my opinion, therefore, those who value the well-
being of their fellow men - the well-being of those who
produce our cars, our aeroplanes, our means of entertainment
and the many articles we use daily and which add to our
comfort - have no option at the present time but to oppose

the calls of antivivisectionists for banning the use of
animals for carcinogenicity tests.   Such a ban now could
ruin any chance of reducing cancer risks to workers as a
result of the implementation of the Health and Safety at
Work Act.

THE RISK OF CANCER FROM SEX HORMONES

        About five years ago, Dr. Herbst and others in the
United States (Herbst et al, 1971, Greenwald et al, 1971)
reported between them 13 cases of a rare form of cancer of
the vagina.   Those affected were all adolescent girls, and
further enquiry revealed that they shared one common feature
in their medical histories: all were the daughters of women
who had been given diethylstilboestrol (DES), a synthetic
sex hormone, in high dosage during pregnancy.   During the
1940's and 1950's, there was a vogue, which started in the
United States and then spread to other countries including
Britain, for treating cases of habitual or threatened
abortion with increasing doses of DES.   Dosing began as
early as the 6th week in pregnancy with doses of 5 mg. per
day, and in some women the daily dose reached 150 mg. per
day by the 35th week of pregnancy, when the treatment was
stopped.   By any criterion, doses of the latter order are
massive, and to-day, in the light of the now recognised
dangers of giving thalidomide and other drugs to pregnant
women, it would be regarded as irresponsible to embark on
such a course of treatment without adequate evidence that
it would not affect the foetus.   Be that as it may, tens
of thousands of pregnant women were treated in this way,
and it is among the daughters of these that otherwise rare
forms of cancer of the vagina and uterine cervix have been
arising.   So far the incidence of such cancers among the
daughters of DES-treated mothers appears to be quite low
(e.g. of the order of 1 in 1,000), and there has been no
excess of any form of cancer among the sons of treated
women.   To date all the cases of vaginal and cervical
cancer have arisen in the United States, and no case has
been seen in Britain, even though a survey by Kinlen and
colleagues (1974) suggested that of the order of 4,500
pregnant women in Britain were treated with DES, mainly
during the 1960's.   There is clear evidence among the
United States series that the risk of vaginal cancer is
highest where exposure to DES began early in pregnancy.

Also, as the most recent study reported by Herbst and his
colleagues (1975) indicates, the vaginal cancers do not
arise out of a clear sky, but against a background of
developmental abnormalities of the genital tract.   Some of
the data from this study are summarised in Table 4.

Table 4.   Frequency of abnormalities in 133 exposed subjects
in relation to week of initiation of diethylstilboestrol
therapy during pregnancy.

Week	Total Number	Vaginal Adenosis(%)	Cervical Erosion(%)	Ridge(%)
8	22	73	100	23
9–12	39	49	92	28
13–16	42	29	81	19
17	30	7	70	13

from Herbst et al, New Engl. J. Med. 334 (1975).

    In the light of these figures, I personally find it
difficult to believe that we will not soon be seeing cases
of vaginal and cervical cancer attributable to prenatal
exposure to DES in this country.   We must, of course, hope
that, as the daughters of DES-treated women grow older, they
will not continue to exhibit an increased risk of these same
or other forms of cancer.   But we have no grounds for
assuming that this will be so, or that their sons will not
be at increased risk of developing one or other form of
cancer.   We know that the incubation period for some kinds
of cancer in humans may be as long as even 50 years.   There
is thus a need to watch these sons and daughters
particularly closely both in their own interests and so that
we can discover as much as possible about the effects of
exposure of humans to DES.   The vaginal and cervical
tumours, which have arisen, are probably indirect
consequences of intrauterine exposure to DES, the primary
effect of hormones being that it interferes with the normal
development of genital tract epithelium.   For reasons not
yet clear, cancer is more likely to develop in abnormal
than in normal genital tract epithelium.

One of the consequences of the recently-discovered risk
of vaginal cancer in the daughters of DES-treated women has
been a reappraisal of the safety of using DES and other sex
hormones in meat-production.   Under certain conditions, the
addition of DES to animal feed, or its implantation into the
ears of beef cattle and sheep, or into the necks of male
chickens, promotes their growth and improves the texture of
the meat produced.   Traces of DES can sometimes be found in
the meat from these animals.   The question is, does the
presence of such traces increase the risk of cancer in those
who eat the meat?   I recently had occasion to survey the
extensive literature on this subject (Roe, 1975), and
concluded to my own satisfaction that the presence of traces
of DES in meat would not increase cancer risk in humans.
There is no reason to believe that, although DES is
synthesised in the laboratory and does not occur in nature,
its effects are in any way different from those of naturally
occurring oestrogens, such as oestradiol-17B.   In high
doses, DES and oestradiol-17B produce almost exactly the
same range of cancers in a range of laboratory animals.
So that, if DES is to be regarded as potentially unsafe in
very low doses, then, to be logical, natural oestrogens must
also be so regarded.   At this point, however, the argument
becomes absurd because all of us here are busy producing
natural oestrogens for the normal functioning of our bodies.
That is even true for the males present for males produce
oestrogens - but in inactive, conjugated forms.   The traces
of oestrogen left in oestrogen-treated meat are small by
comparison with those which we produce in our own bodies.

Hormones, such as oestrogens, are chemical messengers
capable of switching on or off genetic information held in
the nuclei of cells.   If hormones are given in large doses
or over prolonged periods, they can bring about obvious
changes in the body: men given oestrogens develop breasts
and women given androgens grow beards.   Sometimes such
alterations in the body are associated with increases or
decreases in risk of cancer.   Male mice of some strains,
for instance, are extremely apt to develop benign and
malignant tumours of the liver.   In a few strains the
incidence of such tumours reaches 100%, but this figure can
be dramatically reduced by castrating the mice and treating
them with oestrogens.   Similarly, the giving of the male
sex hormones to female mice increases their chances of
developing liver tumours.   In laboratory animals many of

the types of cancer, which are influenced by the administration of sex hormones, are caused primarily by viruses. This is true, for instance, for breast tumours and for leukaemia in mice, both of which occur more frequently when oestrogens are given. At present we have no knowledge concerning viruses which cause cancer in humans. I expect there are some, but their discovery lies in the future. Even when they have been identified, however, it is unlikely that the risk of the kinds of cancer, with which their presence is associated, will be materially altered by doses of sex hormones too low to have any obvious effect on the structure or function of the body.

This brings me to the final matter which merits discussion. Does use of the contraceptive pill affect cancer risk?

It has long been recognised that promiscuity, as well as poor living conditions, are associated with increased risk of cancer of the uterine cervix. During recent years it has been suggested that cancer viruses may be transmitted during sexual intercourse. If this were so, some cases of cervical cancer could be regarded as examples of venereal disease. However this may be, and whatever view any of us hold with regard to the standards of morality of our time, it is clear that promiscuity is rife among the young to-day. The incidence of cancer of the cervix is, therefore, likely to increase during the years to come. The ready availability of contraceptive devices, and particularly of the contraceptive pill, is an important factor that has made possible widespread promiscuity without a concomitant explosion in the birth-rate. During recent years we have learned of some of the undesired effects of the pill, including rare examples of fatal cerebrovascular accident. But the big question that still has not been satisfactorily answered is, "Does taking the pill increase a woman's chances of developing any form of cancer?" The question is, of course, related to the subject we were considering earlier, namely, the development of vaginal cancers in the daughters of women treated with oestrogens during pregnancy. Contraceptive pills contain oestrogens, or substances with related hormonal activity. Moreover, the amounts taken, unlike those present in oestrogen-treated meat, are sufficient to produce physiological effects, e.g., the suppression of ovulation. It is not, therefore, possible to dismiss the question as merely an academic one.

During the past few years two crumbs of relevant information have become available - one of them worrying and the other hopeful.   In 1973, Baum and his colleagues reported 7 cases of a previously rare form of benign tumour of the liver in women who had been taking the pill.   Other workers have seen similar cases.   However, considering the fact that millions of women have been taking contraceptive pills of various formulations for many years, it would seem reasonable to conclude that the liver tumour risk must be very small.

More encouraging is a recent report by Dr. Vessey together with Sir Richard Doll and Miss Keena Jones.   From a comparison of 322 women aged 16 - 45, undergoing treatment for newly diagnosed breast cancer, and 502 matched controls, they found no evidence to suggest that the use of oral contraceptives either increases or decreases the risk of breast cancer.   It is, of course, important to realise, as I pointed out above, that we may eventually find that taking the pill protects some or all women from certain forms of cancer.   We are rightly impatient to know what the truth is, but we have no option but to wait and watch what is happening.   In this particular area, tests on animals are of limited value.   They have already told us that interfering with hormonal status can change cancer risk in either direction.   No animal tests at present available can tell us precisely what changes in cancer risk we can expect to find in women as a result of their taking the pill.

REFERENCES

Baum, J.K., Holtz, F., Bookstein, J.J. and Klein, E.W.
        1973.   Possible association between benign hepatomas
        and oral contraceptives. Lancet 2:926.
Butlin, H.T. 1892.   Cancer of the scrotum in chimney-sweeps
        and others. Brit. Med. J. 1:1341, and, 2:1.
Greenwald, P., Barlow, J.J., Nasca, P.C. and Burnett, W.S.
        1971.   Vaginal cancer after maternal treatment with
        synthetic cestrogens.   New Engl. J. Med. 285:390.
Health and Safety at Work, etc. Act. 1974. HMSO 1975 pp.1-17.
Herbst, A.L., Poskanzer, D.C., Robboy, S.J., Friedlander, L.
        and Scully, R.E. 1975.   Prenatal exposure to
        stilboestrol: a prospective comparison of exposed
        female offspring with unexposed controls.   New Engl.

J. Med. 292:334.
Herbst, A.L., Ulfelder, H. and Poskanzer, D.C. 1971.
    Adenocarcinoma of the vagina: association of maternal
    stilboestrol therapy with tumour appearance in young
    women. New Engl. J. Med. 284:878.
Kinlen, L.J., Badaracco, M.A., Moffett, J. and Vessey, M.P.
    1974. A survey of the use of oestrogens during
    pregnancy in the United Kingdom and of the genito-
    urinary cancer mortality and incidence rates in young
    people in England and Wales. J. Obst. Gynaec. Brit.
    Cwth. 81:849.
Roe, F.J.C. 1975. Carcinogenicity studies in animals
    relevant to the use of anabolic agents in animal
    production. Paper presented at Joint FAO/WHO
    Symposium on the Use of Anabolic Agents in Animal
    Production and its Public Health Aspects, Rome,
    March 17th - 19th, 1975.
Vessey, M.P., Doll, R. and Jones, K. 1975. Oral
    contraceptives and breast cancer: progress report of
    an epidemiological study. Lancet 1:941.

DISCUSSION

Question 1. By what mechanism may industrial or
pharmaceutical chemicals cause cancer to appear?

Answer. Many cancer researchers strive to find
answers to this kind of question and an enormous literature
describes their attempts to do so. It is, however, already
clear that many different kinds of mechanism are involved.
I will mention just four. Firstly, there are chemical
agents which react directly with, or give rise to metabolites
which react directly with cellular nucleic acids and thereby
bring about heritable changes in cells which render them more
likely than normal cells to proliferate as cancers. Certain
constituents of unrefined mineral oils and vinyl chloride
appear to be in this class. Secondly, there are materials
which the body has difficulty in eliminating once they get
into it. The mere physical presence of these materials
over long periods stimulates chronic tissue reactions from
which cancers tend to arise. Asbestos dust appears to
belong to this class. Thirdly, there are agents which do
not alter nucleic acids themselves, but which determine
whether or not genetic information, stored as nucleic acids,
is expressed or not. Such substances may switch on

information relevant to the formation of cancers which
would not otherwise have arisen.   Hormones may act in this
way.   Fourthly, it is thought that cells, which have
suffered alterations in their nucleic acids, such that if
they were able to proliferate they would give rise to cancers,
are prevented from proliferating by immunological mechanisms.
Drugs or other agents which suppress these immunological
defences, have been found to predispose to cancer.   Immuno-
suppressant drugs may also give rise to cancer by permitting
cells infected with cancer viruses to multiply.   Ionising
radiation probably produces cancers by a combination of the
first and fourth of these four mechanisms.

Question 2.   Does social or regional environment show
an influence on the incidence of cancer?

Answer.   Both social and regional factors influence
cancer incidence markedly.   Most authorities believe that
environmental factors generally are far more important than
genetic ones in determining who develops cancers of different
types.   The best evidence that regional environment
influences cancer risk comes from studies on people who
migrate from one region to another.   Provided that the
migrants adopt the social habits of the area into which they
move, the risk of their developing various forms of cancer
is likely to change from the pattern in their region of
origin to the pattern in their new locality.   Moreover, the
change is likely to be more marked the younger they are when
they migrate.

Question 3.   How does age influence the incidence of
cancer?   Are certain age groups more susceptible than
others?

Answer.   The risk of most forms of cancer increases
steeply with increasing age but there are many exceptions.
There are, for instance, some cancers which occur only in
childhood or around the time of puberty.   Also the risk of
developing a tumour of the brain declines in old age.   In
a recent study, Richard Peto and others, including myself,
found that susceptibility to the induction of cancer by a
chemical carcinogen did not increase with age.   Our finding
is consistent with the concept that the increasing risk of
development of many forms of cancer with age is attributable
to the fact that those affected are continuously exposed to

carcinogenic influences and that the unreversed (not necessarily irreversible) effects of such exposure accumulate with age.

Question 4.   What is the effect on the child of progesterone given to the mother throughout pregnancy, starting soon after conception?

Answer.   There have, to my knowledge, been no reports of ill effects on the child.

Question 5.   Is there any evidence that environmental monitoring had reduced carcinogenic risk for people in this country?

Answer.   Improvements in industrial hygiene have certainly greatly reduced risks of cancer among certain groups of workers (e.g. scrotal cancer in cotton spinners and tool setters, mesothelioma and lung cancer in asbestos workers).   It is probable that reduced pollution of air is having a slight effect on lung cancer incidence. Environmental monitoring of other kinds, e.g., seeing that food stuffs are not contaminated to an unacceptable extent with heavy metals, may have reduced cancer risk.   The requirement that drugs, food additives and pesticides should be tested for carcinogenic potential has almost certainly prevented some deaths from cancer.   It is always difficult to give precise answers to questions of this kind because of the impossibility of measuring events which do not happen!

Question 6.   Is there any correlation between the incidence of breast cancer and the use of oral contraception? Also, what is the incidence of breast cancer in those women who have breast-fed their children and those in whom lactation has been suppressed by hormone therapy?

Answer.   The truth is that we have not got enough information yet to know how the use of oral contraception affects breast cancer risk, but there is the encouraging paper recently published in the Lancet by Dr. Vessey and others, entitled, "Oral Contraception and Breast Cancer - Progress Report of an Epidemiological Study."   You will recall from my paper that they found no evidence that the taking of oral contraceptives either increased or decreased the risk of breast cancer.

I shall pass the second part of this question to Mr. Raven.

Answer by Mr. R.W. Raven.   There is no evidence that breast-feeding confers any immunity on the breast against the subsequent development of cancer.   More data are required about the possible adverse effects of suppressing lactation with hormones.

Question 7.   Statistics show there is a decline in the number of people dying from stomach cancer in this country. Can Dr. Roe suggest any reason for this?

Answer.   I think the honest answer is that we simply do not know the reason.   It is very tempting to believe that what people eat has got something to do with it.   It may be because the sort of things ordinary people eat in this country has changed.   The average diet has probably become more nutritious and it may now contain, for instance, more substances that protect in some way against stomach cancer.   However, I think the most likely reason for the improvement is that our food is cleaner - more of us eat more processed food and more of us have refrigerators. We know that certain fungal toxins, such as the one, aflatoxin, that has been found in peanuts, are potent carcinogens.   Whether it can cause cancer of the stomach in man is not known.   It is possible that aflatoxin or other toxins produced by micro-organisms, which contaminate badly stored food, increase the risk of stomach cancer. Support for the view that stomach cancer risk varies with diet comes partly from studies on Japanese migrants.   The incidence of cancer of the stomach in Japan is about five times that in the U.S.A.   When Japanese migrate to the U.S.A. and adopt the eating habits of the indigenous population, their risk of stomach cancer, and particularly that of their children, falls dramatically.

Question 8.   Fifteen years ago before my daughter was born, I had two X-rays, one two months before birth and the second one three weeks before birth.   What are the dangers?

Answer.   This is all 15 years ago and all that we positively know about the effects of X-rays on unborn children, concerns effects up to the age of about 15 years.

The risks are very small; it is only by comparing large
numbers of pregnant women who have been X-rayed and large
numbers of pregnant women who have not been X-rayed that
one can find any detectable difference in cancer risk in
their progeny.   There appears to be a slightly increased
risk of leukaemia in the children of X-rayed women,
especially before the age of 5 years.   Further research on
older children and on larger numbers of children is, in
fact, going on in the Research Department of the Marie Curie
Memorial Foundation at the present time under Dr. Kinnier
Wilson.

        Question 9.   Is there any country in which cancer is
non-existent or has been non-existent?

        Answer.   I think the answer is probably no.   A
Japanese epidemiologist, called Dr. Segi, has collected
information concerning incidences of cancers of various kinds
and sites from 24 countries, for which adequate information
is available.   There is a considerable incidence of cancer
in all these 24 countries, although there are remarkable
differences between the countries in which types of cancer
occur most commonly.   Of course, cancer is a much less
common cause of death in countries where people do not live
long enough to develop the disease.   Wherever the average
age at death is low, one is most unlikely to see a high
incidence of cancer.   Now, there have been reports, usually
in the lay press, of isolated communities in, for instance,
South America or Southern Russia, in which people live to
well over 100 and nobody develops cancer.   There are lots
of snags with this type of information.   Falsification of
age is common and the size of the populations from which the
100+ year-olds have come, cannot be ascertained.   In other
words the collection of very old people, that is seen by
tourists, is a selected group whose rude health and freedom
from cancer is not representative of the whole population of
the area.   I am sure that hopeful observations of this kind
should always be investigated, but one should not be over-
sanguine that some little community has hit upon a way of
being able totally to avoid cancer.

PROGRESS TOWARDS EFFECTIVE COMPUTER SYSTEMS IN MEDICINE

Barry Barber

Director of Operational Research

The London Hospital

There is much in the developing field of medical computing that is relevant to the care and treatment of oncological diseases.   The three particular things that were emphasised by Mr. Raven this morning were research, screening and patient records.   Computers are relevant to all three;   they are also relevant to Dr. Roe's statement that we have no option but to wait and watch since there should be appropriate computer systems included in this waiting and watching.   The setting up of computer systems requires the patience, perseverance and tedious attention to detail that was shown by Marie and Pierre Curie when they isolated radium from pitchblend.

There has been tremendous progress with the development of medical computing systems over the last decade.   Fig. 1 shows a nurse using a ward terminal, rather like a television screen, in a ward at the London Hospital. Almost exactly 10 years ago the London Hospital installed its first computer and had just got its first payroll working.   It was a rather small computer, and ward terminals then were just speculation.   Now there are about 65 terminals in wards and departments of the Hospital and some of these have been operating since the autumn of 1972. The system is normally up and working from 8.00 a.m. until midnight.   This particular nurse has at her fingertips the waiting list for consultants with beds in that ward.   Also, she has basic administrative information for each patient in the ward, and information on the various requests for the microbiology, haematology, biochemistry laboratories, as well as the reports from the microbiology laboratory.   In

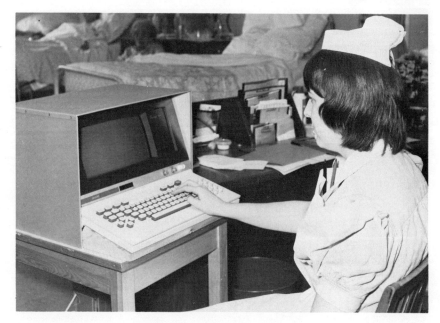

Fig. 1

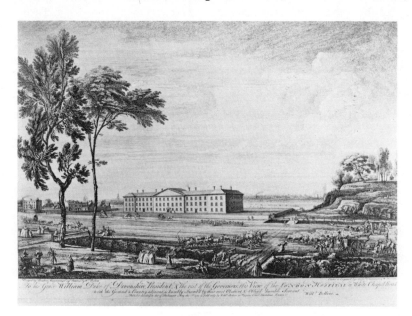

Fig. 2

addition, she can look up the index of patients who have
been admitted, or put on the waiting list, since 1972.
This is quite a transformation in 10 years and it is still
only the first phase of the development.   It is almost as
great a transformation as the present London Hospital is
from the illustration in Fig. 2.   That particular change
took something like 200 years to achieve and we know a
great deal more as a race about urban growth than we do
about computer growth.

   This particular development was made possible by the
initiative taken by the Department of Health and Social
Security in setting up the experimental computer programme
in 1967.   It has placed the United Kingdom in its present
highly developed state in Health Service computing.   The
pioneering work carried out at a number of centres in
designing, operating and utilising advanced computer
systems makes possible the selection and widespread
implementation of major systems during the next decade.
Proper evaluation of the systems already implemented will
enable the Department of Health and the Regional Health
Authorities to plan their computer systems on the basis of
extensive operational experience.

   The attempt to evaluate the computer systems raises
all the fundamental problems of the evaluation of our
Health Care Delivery Systems.   Indeed, it may be that the
concept of the vital role of evaluation will prove more
significant for the Health Service than the introduction
of the computer systems themselves.   The formulation of
systems, objectives and the evaluation of the performance
of the systems against those objectives must be beneficial
and must lead to a better understanding and deployment of
our Health Care Systems.

   The development of computer systems is crucially
important to the development of the monitoring systems
which will facilitate the devolution of decision-making in
the reorganised Health Service to District level.   The
new Department of Health and Social Security planning
system attempts to monitor the functioning of Regions,
Areas and Districts in their provision of health care and
their use of resources.   In this way the allocation of
resources may be more directly related to the provision of
care and in the long run such systems must be simplified,

standardised and computer-based.   Such information systems
and the ability to build computer models of particular
aspects of the health care system are, also, relevant to
the District Health Care Planning Teams.   However, with
all the sophisticated equipment available, computer systems
are still at the stage of the Model T Ford or the gold leaf
electroscope.   It is necessary to exploit the power that
computers provide and concentrate much more on the medical,
nursing and scientific problems, as compared with the
administrative problems that have been considered up to
now.

     Even a cursory look through the 208 pages of the 1974
Annual Review of National Health Service Computing by the
Department of Health and Social Security (1) shows the wide
variety of computing activity within the National Health
Service in the United Kingdom.   The computer systems range
from micro and mini computers to substantial configurations;
the systems range from conventional batch processing to the
most advanced real-time systems supporting over 60 visual
displays.   The applications range from routine financial
and statistical data processing to systems directly
affecting the care of the patients.   Similarly, the
variety of papers presented at the first world conference
on medical informatics, Medinfo 74, in Stockholm in 1974
(2) indicates the volume and diversity of the research and
development activity currently in progress throughout the
world in medical computing.

     Before discussing the computer systems, it is
important to mention the vital research uses of computers.
Mr. Raven's first point related to research.   It must be
appreciated that it is now no longer possible to carry out
extensive research in fields that border on science without
having adequate use of computing facilities.   With proper
facilities, it is possible to do in quite short periods of
time, with relatively little computer experience, much
analysis and data handling that would take months and even
years with manual techniques.   Indeed, this activity
requires wide support and has not been recognised very
clearly in the Health Service, although, of course, the
Universities have recognised this for a long time.
Computer systems, both large and small, are essential
tools for handling statistical analysis, model building,
scientific problem-solving and the analysis of analogue

signals.   Good computing facilities enable research and
development staff to concentrate powerful tools on the
solution of their problems without having to worry about
much of the detail of programming and operating computers.
The requirements for computer systems development and
research using computers are quite different.

DEVELOPMENT OF HEALTH SERVICE COMPUTER SYSTEMS

The development of computer systems is a lengthy
business and the computer world is full of systems that
have failed to achieve satisfactory results.   Brock's
paper (3) provides a salutary and useful analysis of the
reasons why systems fail.   However, there should be no
problems if the systems objectives are clearly perceived
by the prospective users of the computer system and if the
users are fully brought into the design of the system by
the experienced professional computer staff.   In general,
it is desirable to initiate the development with relatively
simple computer systems, building up to the more complex
systems, as the simple systems begin to show benefits and
as staff develop expertise in handling such systems.

Fig. 3 indicates a hierarchy of Health Service Systems,
indicating the lines of development of major systems.
Competence in handling the lower level systems is required
before the more interesting high level systems can be
installed.   Each category of system is discussed in
outline below, but a somewhat fuller discussion is available
in Reference 4.

FINANCE AND ADMINISTRATION SYSTEMS

The first systems to be set up were the financial
systems.   This work provided the basis for the present
Regional Computer Centres and it has developed to include
some aspects of patient administration, such as Hospital
Activity Analysis, as well as certain specialised medical
or scientific data analysis.   By and large this work goes
reasonably well and pays for itself.

The financial systems tend to utilise conventional
batch processing techniques.   Succeeding technical

DEVELOPMENT OF HEALTH SERVICE COMPUTING SYSTEMS

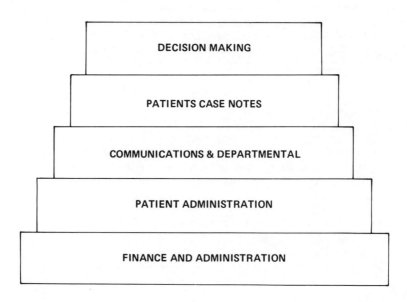

DECISION MAKING

PATIENTS CASE NOTES

COMMUNICATIONS & DEPARTMENTAL

PATIENT ADMINISTRATION

FINANCE AND ADMINISTRATION

Fig. 3

developments are likely to aim towards real-time data input
and file inspection facilities.   The next systems
development will involve a measure of integration between
the financial and the patient administration systems to
provide a revised accounting system allowing budgetary
control to be given to those responsible for the commitment
of resources.   The full integration of these systems will
eventually provide a sensitive means of delegating the
control of the allocation of all Health resources within
the reorganised Service.

PATIENT ADMINISTRATION SYSTEMS

Patient admmnistration was started on small batch
computers taking over from earlier punched card systems to
provide the basic information about hospital workloads.
Although concerned initially with the production of
statistical returns, the data base relates to patient-

orientated information of a mainly administrative kind.
It deals with matters, such as categories of service
provided, the area of residence of the patient, the medical
specialty concerned and the final diagnosis on discharge.
These records are resource-orientated, rather than providing
clinical information such as would appear in the medical
case notes.   Unfortunately, the current batch systems and
the data collection arrangements provide essentially
historic analyses rather than current operational
information.

     Much of the effort of the Department of Health and
Social Security experimental computer programme has been
devoted to the introduction of real-time patient
administration in hospitals and elsewhere.   The basic
functions of patient identification and the collection of
basic administrative information are the essential
preliminaries to medical care.   Such systems are now
routinely operating in a number of centres in the United
Kingdom and elsewhere.   The North Staffordshire Royal
Infirmary have an outpatient administration system which
includes clinic appointments and control.   The London
Hospital has had a real-time waiting list, admission and
discharge system with visual displays on the wards,
operating since 1972.   The Queen Elizabeth Hospital,
Birmingham, also has a patient administration system
developed from earlier work on their previous batch
computer.   The Exeter Community Health Service project
has the beginnings of a community patient administration
functioning.   Often these basic systems also provide some
service of more obviously medical interest and it is
intended to develop the system by including more high level
medical services.

     From a detailed study of the planning and epidemiological
needs of the reorganised Health Service it would seem that
one of the first priorities should be the development of
District and Area wide patient information and index systems
based on the population served.   The first need of the
community physician is to relate the pattern of disease to
the community in which it occurs.   The concept of a master
patient index is discussed at length by Bodenham and Wellman
(5) in their report on "Foundations for Health Service
Management."   One of the major features of the reorganised
Health Service is a change of emphasis towards caring for
a population rather than the management of institutions.

This type of approach in oncology leads directly to a
requirement for a readily accessible national oncological
record system.

COMMUNICATIONS AND DEPARTMENTAL SYSTEMS

The more interesting of these systems appear to
occupy a niche intermediate between the patient
administration systems and the case note systems.   The
system is often concerned with the input of patient
identification and related administrative material and it
often produces output that could, or should, form part of
the patients' case notes.   In between, the system may
produce other outputs related to the internal operation of
the service department such as work sheets, load scheduling,
quality control statistics.   Such systems can be designed
on small computers as strictly limited departmental systems,
or else as hospital wide communications systems which may
ultimately form the basis for an all-inclusive patient case
notes system.   The technical complexity of system design
and implementation escalates rapidly as the systems, and
access to it, becomes more widespread and less department-
orientated.   Collen (6) gives a good summary of the
current progress of hospital information systems while
Stacey and Waxman (7) describe progress on certain limited
problem areas.   Much of the interest in these systems
derives from the desire to make the most of the hospital
resources in expediting the investigation and treatment of
patients.   Such concepts lead naturally to the idea of
scheduling patient care.   The most important application
groups in this section are discussed briefly below.

(a)   Clinical Laboratory Systems

This is a well-proven area of activity and there are a
number of commercially available systems.   The original
impetus for this work arose from the handling of automated
apparatus in the biochemistry laboratory.   Since that time
automated apparatus has spread to the haematology
laboratories and the workloads of all laboratories have
increased immensely, making such systems increasingly
economic and attractive.   Full requesting, reporting and
information retrieval systems have also been integrated

with such laboratory systems.   In addition, requesting and
reporting have been included as part of hospital-wide
communication systems covering other laboratories.   For
instance, the London Hospital implemented a microbiology
system during the spring of 1974 as part of its
communication system which already provided a basic
framework of patient administration.   Some form of
laboratory system should now be regarded as standard
equipment wherever there is a high volume of automated
testing.

(b)   Physiological Monitoring Systems

The most obvious system is that designed to monitor
acutely ill patients in Intensive Care Units or Coronary
Care Units.   Such systems have been operational for many
years and are concerned with capturing appropriate
physiological information.   They are thought valuable in
enabling clinicians to detect trends in the patient's
condition at an early stage and in providing a substantial
data base from which research into the management of the
acutely ill patients may be carried out.   Again, the basic
difficulty is not the technical or of implementing systems
to carry out specified tasks, but the conceptual one of
evaluating the improvements in patient care provided.
Another valuable application relates to the analysis and
reporting of electrocardiograms (e.c.g.), either directly
on line, possibly using the telephone system, or off-line
using some form of magnetic tape storage device.   Such
systems begin to provide computer assistance with
fundamentally medical, as distinct from administrative,
problems.

(c) Radiotherapy Treatment Planning Systems

A variety of programmes have been available to assist
with radiation treatment planning for well over a decade.
This work was developed on a research basis and now a number
of systems are available for use on mini computers.   These
systems are very successful in handling the complex
mathematical calculations involved.   The original hope of
an optimal planning system has proved elusive, but
interactive planning systems are now routine and have proved

extremely valuable.   This application involves the input
of the patient's body contour, the selection and weighting
of certain radiation fields and the repeated modification
of these selections until an acceptable plan is obtained.
The data control is readily handled on a visual display
unit leaving the final field to be printed on a graph
plotter.   In the hands of an experienced treatment
planning technician, good plans may be produced very
rapidly.   This application was the first application for
which an attempt was made to evaluate it within the terms
of Department of Health and Social Security policy on the
evaluation of computer applications.   It was possible (8)
to show criteria for the introduction of such systems on
the basis of effective system running costs and the
treatment planning volume.   The break even point at that
time and for the particular system examined in this case
occurred at about 500 planned patients per year.   If the
radiotherapists justify their clinical requirements in
terms of the planning volume, technological considerations
determine the appropriate system on financial grounds.
(Microfiche copies of this report are still available).

(d)   Automated Health Screening Systems
                and Preventive Medicine

A large number of standard Health Screening Systems
are available, but they have not been widely implemented in
the United Kingdom as a result of the general lack of
enthusiasm for Health Screening.   However, such systems
have had wide application in the United States and elsewhere
and they provide a basis from which some aspects of a mass
preventive medicine service may be initiated.   The major
queries relate to the value of the routine measurements
which may be conveniently automated rather than adequacy of
the associated computer systems.   I hope that the Health
Service will soon be experimenting with such systems.   I
have long seen an effective outpatient investigation centre
as a link between the community and the hospital service.
Such a centre would need effective computer systems, not
only for data capture and analysis on a large scale, but
also for communication with the primary care teams and the
hospital staff.   The patient flows would be organised as
shown in Fig. 4.   The appropriate development of
oncological screening systems was emphasised as Mr. Raven's
second point.

THE DELIVERY OF MEDICAL CARE

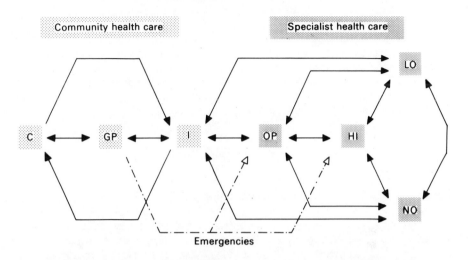

C Citizen GP Family Doctor I Outpatient investigation OP Specialist Consultation
HI,LO,NO Residential Accommodation with High/Medium, Low, No Nursing & Medical Care

Fig. 4

The major Health Service computer applications currently in this category relate to the local authorities' vaccination and immunization programmes, which were pioneered in West Sussex and have been exceedingly successful in improving the coverage of these services. Such systems have been shown to be, not only effective in improving the service, but also cost-effective.   It is expected that the reorganisation will lead to an increase in these activities in preventive medicine.

(e)   Other Departmental and Communications Systems

A wide variety of other systems have been pioneered or are under development, but have not yet reached the stage of being transferable to other centres or commercially

available.   These include systems dealing with X-ray
requesting, reporting and departmental organisation,
nursing records for patients and work scheduling, nursing
staff records and manpower planning, pharmacy stock control,
drug prescribing and such like.   In addition, a number of
specialised systems are available, such as those for
handling gamma camera data analysis for diagnostic use with
radioactive isotopes.   References previously quoted (2 and
6) gives much fuller coverage of such work.

NEXT DEVELOPMENTS

From Fig. 3 it is clear that I expect that the next
steps will involve the development of case notes systems,
and this brings me to Mr. Raven's third point.   The work
done so far is merely preliminary to the more interesting
and intellectually rewarding medical decision-making systems
that will ultimately be built.   The case notes systems will
provide accurate data input for such sophisticated systems
as well as being valuable in their own right.   In 1968 when
the basic decisions were taken on the London Hospital project
it was thought that the construction of a case notes system
was beyond our reach.   However, with current technology
and the experience of the existing systems, I believe that
such systems could be built.   Indeed, a number of centres
are beginning to make progress in this area (e.g. Weed: 9)
although the systems seem to be rather expensive at the
present time.   It might be that development in one segment
of medicine might prove a more fruitful way of approaching
the problem than attempting to tackle the complete range of
medical activity.   This does not necessarily mean that the
computer system will attempt to duplicate the familiar
scribbled patient case notes; computer case notes will be
structured and logical (e.g. ref. 10).   Also, it may be
some while before operational systems are widely accepted.
However, computer case summaries can readily be designed
for a a variety of purposes.   The major difficulty is that
of getting the material into the computer accurately,
reliably and without undue delay.   At the London Hospital
this has been done with obstetric summaries by having a
computer coding form as the centre to the manual case notes.
It is filled up during the patient's care and sent to the
computer centre on discharge.   The letter to the general
practitioner is produced for issue by the computer from the
computer case record.   The letter is then checked and

signed by the relevant medical staff.

Computer systems must be used and found useful; otherwise they merely become an accumulation of useless and inaccurate material.

Many cancer registration schemes use computing facilities for the analysis of basic computer records, and there is no doubt that these records could be expanded to provide a full summary of the patient's care. The main requirement is that the information should be analysed and utilised locally, regionally and nationally. At present, the data collection systems appear more concerned with the incidence of oncological diseases than with the effectiveness of treatment. It would seem highly desirable to scrutinise the performance of the various centres in their treatment of different types of disease in order to draw tentative conclusions about the relative merits of various types of treatment. It is clear that this analysis can only yield tentative conclusions to be subjected to the discipline of controlled clinical trials, but nevertheless it would begin to focus attention on the basic question of interest to the patients and clinicians alike: "What is the best treatment for specific diseases at specific sites at specific stages?" Such systems could be based on batch processing computers at the Regional computer centre, but it would probably be better to develop them on small local computers with a few terminals at key points throughout an Oncology Centre. The terminals could be used to enter relevant information into some form of structured case notes throughout the patient's period of care and follow-up. The design must suit the needs of the medical staff, providing the right information, at the right time, in the right place and in the right form - as well as collecting accurate data in the first place.

They could be readily designed and implemented at individual centres. However, it would be much more economical if a national design study was set up in conjunction with the relevant professional organisations to specify a system that could be implemented rapidly nationwide once it had been rendered operational at the development site.

The key requirements are basic agreement about the minimum data to be collected, ease of data capture and

compatibility with other national data collection systems.
Experience with computing systems has shown that small self-
contained schemes can be implemented much faster than large
multi-purpose systems.   This proposed system might, therefore,
be rendered **operational** at an early date and provide useful
data for the development of oncology in this country.   In
addition, it would provide valuable computer experience for
the development of other systems in oncology and other
patient record systems in medicine.   In some senses the
reorganisation of the Health Service opens up all sorts of
possibilities and the development of oncological case notes
systems would appear to be one of the possibilities that
should be explored - possibly on a Regional basis from the
Regional oncology centre.

REFERENCES

1. Annual Review of National Health Service Computing, 1974.
        Parts 1 and 2.   Department of Health and Social
        Security.
2. Medinfo 74.   First World Conference on Medical
        Informatics.   Stockholm 5 - 10, August, 1974.
        Papers edited Anderson, J. and Forsythe, J.M.,
        Almqvst and Wiksell, Uppsala, Sweden, 1974.
3. "What went wrong?   An analysis of mistakes in data
        processing," Brocks, B.J., 1969, September.
        Accountancy, 666.
4. Computer Information Systems in Health Care: a series
        of six lectures based on Swedish and British
        experience.   Symposium held in Moscow, February,
        1975.   pub. Sperry Univac.
5. Foundations for Health Service Management: a Scicon
        report for the Scottish Home and Health Department
        on the requirements for a health service information
        system.   Bodenham, K. and Wellman, F.   Nuffield
        Provincial Hospitals Trust, Oxford University Press,
        London, 1972.
6. Hospital Computer Systems: how to use computers in
        medical centers for better patient care. Collen, M.F.
        John Wiley and Sons, New York, 1974.
7. Computers in Biochemical Research, Vol. IV, Stacey, R.W.
        and Waxman, B.D.   New York Academic Press, 1974.
8. Computerised Dose Computational, a report prepared by the
        British Institute of Radiology and the Department

of Health and Social Security.   Barber, B., the
London Hospital, 1973.
9.   The Problem-Orientated Medical Record:
(Supplement to reference 10)
1. Operating Manual for Computer System
2. An Atlas of Physical Examination Abnormalities
3. The Computer and Medical Education
Problem-Oriented Medical Information Systems
Laboratories, Cleveland Metropolitan General
Hospital, School of Medicine, Cape Western Reserve
University, Cleveland, Ohio, U.S.A.
10. Medical Records, Medical Education and Patient Care,
Weed, L.L.   Chicago, Press of Cape Western
Reserve University, 1971.

DISCUSSION

Question 1.   Does the use of computer systems affect
confidentiality?

Answer.   The answer is that obviously it does, but
there is no reason why one should not make the computer
systems much more secure than, for instance, the pile of
case notes one may find in hospital basements, odd corridors
and secretaries' offices.   Confidentiality could be very
much better and one would hope in the reorganised service,
as notes are required throughout Districts, that we shall
make self-conscious efforts to ensure the confidentiality
of this material.

Question 2.   Owing to the failure of computers to work
out correct pay for staff, is there a fail-safe system in
use when using computers for radium treatment?

Answer.   Obviously all technology has to be used
sensibly.   The reasons why computers get the wrong answers
are twofold.   In the first case the programme may be wrong
or in error in some way and, in the second case, it may
have been fed with the wrong data.   In any well-designed
system, programme errors are sorted out and eliminated at
an early stage;   so any system that is put into even
administrative use, let alone medical use, should have had
these problems eliminated during the testing period.   From
there, one has to make sure that the right information goes

in.   If, for instance, you are trying to do some treatment
planning and you insist on putting data for conventional
250 KV beams into it when you really meant the information
for linear accelerators or Cobalt beams, you cannot expect
to get the right answer.   Similarly, in converting to S.I.
Units, as we are currently being encouraged to do, if you
insist on ignoring the difference between millimols and
milliEquivalents or between inches and centimetres, you
cannot expect accurate results.

Question 3.   Since so much valuable data about patients
with cancer is currently being lost because of poor
documentation, what suggestions have you to make to rectify
this situation?

Answer.   The most obvious suggestion, and it follows
from the papers read by Mr. Raven, Dr. Roe and myself, is
for something that looks like a national cancer case notes
system, that can be handled by computers and thus be
properly analysed.   A vast amount of observational data is
being lost, and this is probably the only way that one can
get hold of it effectively.

CANCER EDUCATION AND TRAINING - MEDICAL

R.A. Sellwood

Professor of Surgery

University Hospital of South Manchester

Although we hear and read a great deal about the need
to educate the public about cancer, much less emphasis is
placed on the educational needs of doctors and nurses whose
knowledge of the disease is frequently incomplete, and whose
attitudes are often unduly pessimistic.

In an experiment at the Christie Hospital, Manchester,
the attitudes of the medical and nursing professions to
malignant disease was studied by asking family doctors,
students and nurses the following question: "Of 100
middle-aged people with the following diseases, how many
would you expect to be alive and well five years after
appropriate treatment?" The diseases listed were early
cancer of the larynx, breast and cervix, early seminoma of
the testis and early Hodgkin's disease. Early laryngeal
cancer has a five year survival rate of 75% but 80% of
those questioned gave a wrong answer. A majority gave an
answer of 50%, and a considerable proportion (30 - 40%)
thought only a quarter of the patients survived for five
years. This terrible pattern of pessimism emerged for all
the diseases listed and was consistent for the three groups
of individuals tested. Because of these depressing
results, a positive effort was made to teach students the
true outcome of the treatment of cancer; and over a three
year period this was stressed in their lectures and
tutorials. When they were re-examined after this period
of teaching, the results, instead of improving, had become
worse, with again a marked pessimistic leaning. It seems
clear, at least in Manchester, that the people who more

103

than anyone else must influence public thinking about the
disease, often do not know the answers to simple questions
about cancer, and are unduly pessimistic about the outcome
of treatment.   One way to change the attitudes of doctors
to cancer might be to introduce into the curriculum of
medical schools a course on oncology, similar to the courses
most students now receive in other major specialities.

The problems of medical education are, however, much
broader than this, and in recent years the medical profession
as a whole has become conscious of the need to teach and
learn oncology.   With this in mind, the British Association
of Surgical Oncology was formed two years ago and it now has
over 300 members drawn from every walk of surgical life.
They include very junior surgical trainees and very senior
members of the profession from a variety of different
disciplines.   One function of the Association is to
formulate ideas about surgical education in oncology, for
established surgeons and for surgeons in training.   In
Britain most cancers are and will continue to be treated in
district general hospitals by general surgeons with a wide
range of interests.   Their needs must be our first priority
when we choose topics and select papers for meetings.   Most
important of all is our responsibility to those young
surgeons who wish to make their career in oncology.   It is
encouraging that so many of them have sought advice from the
Association about their training and that the work presented
by them at our meetings has been of such high calibre.
Clearly we are obligated to establish nationally suitable
programmes of training to cater for their needs.

Although there is a healthy disagreement about detail,
the principles, on which training should be based, are
agreed and may be defined as follows.

1.   The surgical oncologist must have received a
broadly based training in general surgery and hold a
Fellowship in one of the Royal Colleges of Surgeons.

2.   His programme of higher specialist training must
be sufficiently flexible to enable him to choose ultimately
between a career as an oncologist in one of the oncological
centres or as a general surgeon with a special interest in
oncology in a district general hospital.

3.   No single hospital or institute can train an oncologist.   He must receive the breadth of surgical experience which can be acquired best in a district general hospital and a special experience in depth which is available only in the major centres.

4.   No trainee can be expected to acquire all the special skills which constitute oncology but each must receive training in two or three special fields, for example, head and neck oncology, breast cancer, paediatric oncology and pelvic oncology.

5.   Each trainee must receive a special experience of chemotherapy, radiotherapy and the surgical pathology of malignant disease.   This experience must be provided in a clinical situation and not in a classroom.

6.   Facilities for cancer research must be available to all, and an opportunity provided for a period in full time research if required.

Three centres, Leeds, Manchester and Southampton have produced detailed programmes of training which fulfil the criteria proposed by the Association, and others, including the Royal Marsden Hospital and associated hospitals in the South West Metropolitan Region have programmes in preparation. Several of the London undergraduate teaching hospitals, including Charing Cross, King's College, St. Mary's, University College and the Westminster Hospitals will provide unique experience and facilities and many district general hospitals throughout Britain have agreed to make a contribution.

Research is an essential part of training and it is relevant to ask certain questions about the distribution of our resources.   At present much research is carried out on rats and mice with tumours which bear no relationship to human tumours histologically, and which behave clinically in a quite different way.   In recent years only one quarter of the papers published in the British Journal of Cancer have been about human cancer;   does this mean that only a quarter of the resources available for cancer research are spent on human cancer?   Perhaps this is an overstatement, but it raises the questions of whether it is right to deploy resources in this way, and what dividends have been achieved by such work?

In summary, it seems that it is necessary to provide better educational programmes for students if their present pessimistic attitudes to cancer are to be changed. In surgery, steps are being taken to improve educational standards and hopefully this in turn will produce better educators. Finally, it is important to ask whether cancer research, which is an important part of education, is being carried out in the best possible way.

REFERENCE

"Cancer and the Problem of Pessimism," by Eric Easson.
    Ca. 1967, Volume 17, No. 1.

DISCUSSION

Question 1. If a patient asks outright if he has cancer, should he be told the truth or should the truth be evaded? What benefits could be gained by patients having a knowledge of the truth? Why are many doctors reluctant to inform cancer patients and their relatives of their condition? How well informed are patients about their disease when they come to the doctor?

Answer. I am surprised that three of those five questions come from Ward Sisters. They really ought to know perfectly well that there are no rules about what you say to an individual patient. Each of them is different and you have to use your judgment about what you say to them. Now, with experience, one makes less mistakes, but I am quite sure that I am sometimes over-frank with patients and sometimes I am not frank enough. Hopefully, with more experience I will do better, but the fact remains, it is an individual decision for the individual doctor about the individual patient and you just cannot lay down rules and regulations about what you say to people.

Question 2. Do statistics exist on the successful treatment of cancer?

Answer. Yes. Mr. Burn presented quite a lot of them and so did I.

Question 3.   Whenever I ask women doctors about their regular smears, they confess they do not have them.   Why is this?

Answer.   It is a well known phenomenon that the medical profession do not believe they are as other men or women as the case may be.

CANCER EDUCATION AND TRAINING - NURSING

Robert Tiffany

Head of the Department of Nursing Studies

Royal Marsden Hospital, London and Surrey

The need for more education and training for nurses in oncology has become increasingly evident over the past few years. For some time many nurse educators have felt concerned about the small amount of attention given to this subject during the nurse's basic training, but it is, of course, very difficult in a three-year work-learn programme to prepare nurses adequately to meet all the demands expected of them as registered nurses. As the patterns of health care change, nursing education has had to accommodate itself to meet these changes; so the nurse now in training has to have a much wider background than was previously required. Mental health, obstetrics, geriatrics, community-care options give the nurse a much wider background to care, but limit to some extent the depth of knowledge in any one speciality. Medical specialization and the multiplicity of specialist units have meant that during basic training it is impossible to prepare nurses adequately for all the situations in which they may later find themselves. What we can do, and what is being done, is to lay down firm foundations on which we can build the basic principles of nursing care so that our newly-qualified nurses are adaptable and capable of changing from one working situation to another without unnecessary trauma, which is so essential in our rapidly-changing and increasingly technologically-orientated society.

As the need for post-basic training has been increasing, it can no longer be looked upon as a luxury for the privileged few but should rather be considered as an essential part of professional development if we are to maintain and improve our standards of patient care.

To meet these increasing demands for post-basic
education and to standardize nationally the curriculum of
training the Joint Board of Clinical Nursing Studies was
established in 1969.   Their prime function was to decide
priorities in continuing nurse education, and, although the
Board was very much orientated to the hospital service
during its first term of office, it was given new "terms of
reference" to extend into the health services in general.
Courses were planned and a schedule of specialities for
consideration drawn up.   These were to be examined from
the point of view of urgency and with regard to manpower
planning.   They decided that a course in cancer nursing
was needed, and in 1973 a specialist panel was set up to
produce an outline curriculum.   This was approved in 1974.

At the present time the Royal Marsden Hospital is the
only centre operating this approved course, but it is hoped
that other centres will be commencing courses before the
end of 1975.   These courses are based to a large extent on
courses previously arranged by individual specialist
hospitals, which have been running for several years, but
we now have the advantage of a nationally-agreed curriculum
and a method of certification of successful course members
acceptable to all hospitals, and, therefore, giving the
standardization so necessary in these days of high labour
mobility.

The content of the course is designed to cover all
aspects of oncology, and on completion of the course we hope
to have a nurse who is knowledgeable and skilled in all
aspects of care relating to malignant disease, who shows an
attitude as optimistic towards cancer as a curable disease
as towards any other disease and who recognises the value
and contribution which the various types of treatment make
to the cure of cancer, and that where cancer is not curable
valuable palliation may be achieved.

Nurses undertaking this course, which lasts for six
months, have five weeks formal teaching based on a block
system of lectures, supplemented by ward tutorials and
clinical teaching.   Clinical experience is gained in
radiotherapy, surgery, medical oncology and a speciality of
their choice, such as terminal care, paediatrics or

outpatients' department.   During this time, students are
encouraged to participate in ward rounds and unit meetings
to discuss specific patient treatment and care.   Students
are also encouraged to attend the conferences of the various
medical divisions which are relevant to their clinical work,
and visits to units and departments, whose work has a direct
bearing upon patient care and management are arranged in the
course of their clinical experience.

It is necessary in any specialist subject that the
student should understand the subject in depth and the
course is, therefore, of a high academic standard.
Throughout the course students are assessed by a series of
objective-type tests, they must submit a series of essays
and a project for their final examination, and a continual
assessment is made of their practical skills.

The material covered by the course includes: the
nature of cancer, carcinogenesis and the environmental
factors relating to malignant disease, methods of detection,
the principles of treatment, and the specific needs of the
different age groups, including children.

During the course we hope that our students will begin
identifying patients' problems and assessing their needs,
and that they will be able to provide resources and
facilities to meet individual physical, social and spiritual
needs.   Our aim is to return the patient to society as
independent as possible and, therefore, an understanding of
the principles of rehabilitation and the role the nurse can
play in supporting other members of the caring professions,
such as physiotherapists and social workers, is essential
in helping the patient to deal with any defects that he may
have as a result of his disease or treatment.   We have been
fortunate in having the experienced advice of the
Rehabilitation Officer of the Marie Curie Memorial
Foundation in planning this particular part of our programme.

Patients to-day are quite rightly demanding to be better
informed about their illness.   Fortunately, we are moving
away from the old argument as to whether or not to tell the
patient that he has cancer.   The question now is rather how
to tell him.   Of course, communication does not mean that
the doctor has had a chat with the patient.   It implies
that the patient has understood and is aware of the

consequences of any decision taken regarding his care.
During this period the patient can be helped immensely by
nurses skilled in communication and in establishing good
relationships with the patient and his family.   We hope
that, through training, our nurses will be aware of the
influences of verbal and non-verbal communication and the
effects of breakdown in communication.   In developing
human relationship skills, we trust that the nurses will
become sensitive to cues given by patients and their
families regarding their individual needs and fears.

It seems safe to assume that the more sophisticated
the patient is about his role, the more likely he is to
facilitate the roles of the various people engaged in his
therapy.   By viewing the patient as a participating member
of the treatment team, instead of a passive recipient of
our care, he will become involved to a great extent as a
helpful and knowledgeable person in the planning and
management of his illness and in the specific elements of
his care.

In caring for patients with persistent malignant
disease, cancer hospitals have had an advantage and a
disadvantage over general hospitals.   For so long many
nurses have thought of cancer hospitals as terminal-care
homes or, at their best, homes for the incurable.
Attitudes towards the care of a patient are changing and a
much more optimistic view is now expressed.   We have been
able to gain some advantages from past pessimism in the
care of our terminal patients.   The nursing-care plans
and policies for this group of patients within our cancer
hospitals are probably more advanced than in any other
sphere of medicine.   Not that our patients need better
care - to observe patients dying from neuro-muscular
disorders or chronic bronchitis reminds us that their needs
are often far greater than those of the cancer patient -
but we have been able to set standards for this type of
care that can be modelled by other specialities.   In
training our nurses for this particular type of care, we
stress the importance of encouraging the patient and helping
him to develop and maintain the maximum capacity for normal
living and obtaining the fullest quality of life.   We also
stress the importance of preserving the dignity of the
patient and the acceptance of the inevitability of death.
Death should be looked upon not as a failure of our
treatment but rather as the completion of our care.

No course of study for nurses to-day would be complete
without reference to management training, and, of course,
some training in the skills of ward and unit administration
is essential, for many of our course members will, on
completion of the course, leave to take senior nursing
appointments.   In this part of their syllabus, however,
our main concern is with training for the management of
patient care;   how to form nursing assessments of patients;
to make individual goals and objectives for patients that
are measurable and attainable;   how to plan a patient's day
and his clinical care during that period, and the over-all
nursing plan leading to his discharge home to his family,
or into the care of the community services.

We hope to give our students an understanding of the
basic methods of learning and teaching and they should be
able to impart these necessary skills and knowledge
effectively to patients, relatives and staff.   Teaching
the patient to care for himself is the most effective
nursing procedure, and teaching relatives is of equal
importance.   It is a tragedy that we still find to-day
patients discharged home with a colostomy and the first
time their family sees it is at home when a crisis arises.
How much better to teach wives and husbands to care for
their spouse's colostomy during the period of hospitalization
when any fears and anxieties can be expelled.

To maintain the professional standards of nursing, an
understanding of the principles of basic research and
clinical-research methods is desirable.   Nursing to-day
cannot be based solely on the traditions of the past.   We
must be able to evaluate our practices and procedures,
develop new procedures and techniques and give an evaluation
of new equipment and materials.   If we are to improve our
present standards of nursing care, it must be achieved by
constantly reviewing our present care systems and an
appreciation of research methods is valuable in making an
objective assessment of alternative nursing-care programmes.

To summarize the aims and objectives of post-basic
training in oncological nursing, we hope to achieve a
standard of care for our patients that is in keeping with
rapid developments and improvements in medical technology.
Our nurses should be skilled in caring for patients
receiving all modalities of therapy and be sensitive to the

needs of patients and relatives in planning and carrying
out nursing-care policies.   When staff are well trained
and prepared to undertake this type of nursing, it can be
one of the most exciting and rewarding areas of nursing
activity.

Not all nurses who are caring for cancer patients,
will be able to attend such courses, and this is
understandable, for most cancer patients are cared for in
general hospitals, or in the community, where the nursing
of cancer patients forms only a part of the nurse's total
responsibility.   To meet the needs of this group of nurses,
several programmes have been arranged.   Regular symposia
on topics, such as Head and Neck Tumours, Paediatric Oncology,
Genito-Urinary Tumours, Gastro-Intestinal Tumours, are
arranged to enable nurses working in these fields to be kept
up-to-date with current trends in cancer treatment as applied
to their own speciality.   The move towards greater community
care, coupled with better control of malignant disease, has
meant an increase in the number of cancer patients being
cared for by the community nursing services.   To meet the
needs of these nurses, a series of two-day workshops have
been arranged by the Royal Marsden Hospital in co-operation
with the Queen's Institute of Nursing and Chiswick
Polytechnic.   These deal with the domiciliary care of the
cancer patient.   At present these workshops are attended
by experienced district nurses, district nurses in training
and some hospital-based nurses to give them an insight into
community-care problems, but we hope soon to make them
inter-disciplinary sessions for all members of the primary
health-care team.   The health visitor plays an important
role in health education and to enable her to be kept
informed of current developments a series of study days
have been held during the past two years.   The need for a
more positive approach to health education in relation to
cancer has become increasingly evident.   To facilitate
this, we have arranged to hold one-week refresher courses
for health visitors.   This is a joint venture between the
Royal Marsden Hospital and the Council for the Education
and Training of Health Visitors, and the courses will
commence in September, 1975.

Finally, we return to the problem of better education
for the student nurse during her basic training.   At the
Royal Marsden Hospital during 1975 we shall be meeting
over 1,000 student nurses from twenty co-operating hospitals

for study days specializing in the care of the cancer
patient.

In this paper I have tried to give an outline of the
need for continuing education in oncology for nurses to
enable us to give effective therapeutic and supporting
care.   I have described the work being done at the Royal
Marsden Hospital, in co-operation with other professional
bodies, to meet these needs, but, of course, similar work
is being undertaken by nursing-education departments of
other cancer centres throughout the country.   I am
grateful to the Marie Curie Memorial Foundation for giving
me the opportunity to discuss our plans and policies with
such a distinguished audience, and my department would be
grateful for any comments you may wish to make, or any
advice that you may wish to give us.

DISCUSSION

Question 1.   Has Nursing Oncology now emerged as a
distinct entity?

Answer.   Oncology is now well established as a
medical speciality and it is a natural progression that
specialist nursing should develop along similar lines.
The value of having trained nursing experts to share in the
management of cancer patients enables us to give the best
possible service to the patient and support to the patient's
family.

Question 2.   I should be interested to learn what
kind of help can be given to the patient and relatives on
the return of the patient to home after a period in an
Intensive Care Unit or after a major operation for cancer.

Answer.   I think that many kinds of help can be given
to the patient who has been returned home following a
period of intensive care for radical cancer surgery.

Firstly, we should consider being more honest with
our patients.   At present it is common practice in many
centres to avoid the problem of honest discussion with the
patient, any discussions being confined to the patient's
relatives.   This can only produce a situation of stress

within the family, which is so evident to staff working in
the community services.   A better approach would be to
have more open discussions with patients and relatives
together before discharge and at follow-up clinics.   Often
the attitude of "The patient does not want to know" is a
rationalization of "I do not like to tell" and the problem
may lie more with the therapist than with the patient.

Another area is the altered body image that may be the
result of cancer surgery.   Such obvious procedures as
radical mastectomy and the creation of a stoma come easily
to mind.   We live in a society in which sexuality plays a
prominent part.   This should be considered before
discharging patients back into the community.   The nurse
can play a valuable role in assessing the anxieties and
fears that may be present with the patient and her/his
partner, and, by counselling, reduce the psychological
trauma that may follow radical mutilating surgery.

Question 3.   I shall shortly be in charge of nursing
services for a brand new Cancer Unit.   What qualities do I
look for when recruiting staff and what services should I
try to initiate when forming the policies for the Continuing
Care Unit?

Answer.   The qualities I should look for in starting
a cancer unit would be similar to those in any hospital unit,
with particular emphasis on maturity, sympathy and an ability
to deal with the emotional needs of patients and their
families.

In forming the policies for a continuing care unit, it
is essential to have clearly defined channels of communication
between all members of the caring team.   A multidisciplinary
approach to all unit problems is vital and the involvement of
the patient and his family in planning individual aspects of
care should be established practice.

Question 4.   Do you think it would be practicable for
nursing schools to run simplified nursing courses for the
lay public as an aid to families who have to care for
patients in the community?

Answer.   No.   I think it is important that families
should be instructed in the care of patients discharged into
the community.   This, however, should be undertaken

primarily in the hospital, before discharge, as part of the
nursing-care policy on the ward.   After discharge,
education should be re-inforced and extended by the community
health services, who can adapt the teaching to particular
home circumstances.

Question 5.   What steps can be taken to give cancer
education and training more prominence in the nursing
curriculum?

Answer.   Cancer education is already included in the
nursing curriculum.   The difficulty arises in the
interpretation by individual schools of nursing as to the
time given to this subject and the depth in which it is
explored.

Question 6.   Do you think there is a role for the
Clinical Nurse Specialist in Oncology?

Answer.   Yes.   I think there is a need for specialist
nurses in oncology to undertake the various aspects of care
related to the differing modalities of therapy.   This
specialist nurse should function as a consultant member of
the health-care team at hospital and community levels.

Question 7.   How do you think the role of the nurse
could be extended in oncology and do you consider this a
good thing?

Answer.   If we are to maintain and extend the
treatments available to cancer patients and increase the
number of diagnostic investigations available, these will
inevitably have to be undertaken by members of the nursing
profession.   The introduction of the stoma therapist has
dramatically improved the standard of care given to stoma
patients.   The introduction of I.V. therapy nurses and the
extended use of nurses in diagnostic centres has meant an
increase in the number of patients able to receive prompt
treatment, which is a vital component of cancer control.

CANCER EDUCATION AND TRAINING - MEDICAL SOCIAL WORK

Joyce Bardsley

Senior Social Worker
Christie Hospital and Holt Radium Institute
Manchester

When I was asked originally to speak at this meeting, I panicked and felt I could not possibly do it. I had worked on the radiotherapy unit for only a year and doubted my ability. However, I discussed this with colleagues and realised that, although my experience in this particular hospital was of short duration, I have been working with cancer patients for many years. There are, of course, a very high percentage of patients treated for the condition, who never actually get to radiotherapy units, and more people are cared for and die at home than either in radiotherapy units or in special care units which are established in various parts of the country; so there is a store of knowledge not actually associated with those treating malignant disease alone.

When I transferred from general hospital to the radiotherapy hospital, I was struck by the very different attitudes to the disease - attitudes as different as the poles in a magnet. In the general hospital referrals were all accompanied by the pursed mouth, raised eyebrow and a general air of pessimism - all very negative feelings. In the radiotherapy unit the attitude is positive - that patients have come to be treated for a condition which can either be cured or controlled, and even at worst and when there is little that can be done in this way, palliative measures are attempted, and pain and death are something to be fought to the last ditch. Social workers, working every day in close proximity to malignant disease, have somehow to get over this attitude to others working in general hospitals, and particularly to those working in the

community.   I feel the first thing we must do is to
educate others into the idea that the word, "cancer," is
generic.   It covers many conditions, some of which are
curable, others can be controlled;   just as the term,
"rheumatism," covers many types of illness.   Incidentally,
the most painracked, physically tortured people I have seen
are those who have had to live many years with arthritis
and to go on living with it - not anybody with cancer.
Social workers should be taught, as part of their training,
more about illness.   There must be more willingness on our
part to share whatever knowledge we have with others,
especially those who are seeing malignant disease away from
the hospital setting.   We must try to teach some kind of
rational and perspective that of all diseases and conditions
cancer is not necessarily the worst one with which one can
be afflicted, and there are many occasions when the
prognosis is much better than in other diseases.

     At the present time I have a patient who had a radical
mastectomy and radiotherapy.   She has, allied to this, a
severe heart condition and pulmonary embolism.   Her breast
gives her no problems.   Her heart causes her much pain and
distress.   In geriatric cases when trying to get Part III
accommodation, there is usually an inclination to put the
patient into a home for the terminally ill, even though the
disease is not the main problem, and the greater issues for
concern are mainly of old age.   Whether this will still
apply when we have Part III accommodation to spare, it is
difficult to say.   I think attitudes will remain the same.
There is a kind of taboo, almost a feeling of pornography,
towards patients with malignant disease.   This applies
very much to medical and nursing staff, as well as to the
relatives of patients.   Medical and nursing staff are
usually reluctant to tell patients that they have this
condition and relatives themselves are very often terrified
that patients should be told the diagnosis.   We must break
these taboos.   As social workers we can help to do this,
but first we must put our own house in order, and I believe
that those of us working with the condition, have certain
responsibilities to educate, interpret and advise outside
agencies.

You know, there is a kind of mystique about hospital and medical matters, which we have got to be prepared to break down. We must talk to patients in the language which they can understand, and stop using jargon, and, though I am sure that at each stage of the proceedings, nurses and doctors do tell patients what is happening, people who are frightened, bewildered in a strange environment, do not always hear what is said. We must explain, if necessary, again and again what is happening. We in hospital must be prepared to explain to community workers what exactly is happening to patients and the techniques that are being carried out. I am constantly having to explain to others that E.U.A. and cystoscopy are not treatments, but only a way of seeing properly exactly how a condition in a somewhat inaccessible site is or is not progressing.

One young community social worker telephoned me in a heated manner about the fact that an elderly gentleman, who received a home help once a week, had been discharged two days after an operation and had not been sent to convalesce. She had not been notified and more home help had not been asked for. When I investigated, it was a patient who came in quite regularly, or, as he termed it, "bed and breakfast;" he was not worried and could not wait to get home. The anxiety here was generated completely by the worker - somebody who had no knowledge of the procedures involved and was terrified of her own feelings about cancer - and was NOT generated by the patient. We managed to divert this before her feelings were put onto her patient and all was well. Many workers, who have not had the experience of hospital, or the trauma of diagnosis, have not themselves come to terms with illness, particularly those which may be fatal. I feel this is very sad and we in hospital must be prepared to take more students and be involved more in social work training, taking part in seminars in service training programmes. It is, after all, the people at community level, who are dealing with the day to day problems which illness brings. This applies not only to social workers, but to health visitors and to district nurses. I am always dismayed by the pessimistic way that district nurses view malignant diseases.

One thing that surprised me when I went to a cancer treating hospital was the amount of practical help that we are able to get for our patients: cancer is a very emotive word.   People are willing to give time and money to helping those with the condition.   This is good, but we must be prepared to help all our colleagues to get it for their patients by advising them of the sources and resources available.   At the present time I am having a discussion with a community worker who wants me to apply to a cancer fund for £160 to send a family to a camp for a holiday. Two years ago the father was treated for a stage 1 carcinoma of the antrum and his response to treatment was good; he is back at work.   This problem family, or family with problems, whichever way you put it, have been known first to children's departments, then to social services for some seven years, long before the father was diagnosed.   The worker thinks a holiday would help and the comparatively wealthy cancer fund as good a way as any to get the money for this.   He got annoyed when I asked him what way the father's condition had exacerbated the problems within the family.   He acknowledged the fact that it had not but it had brought a degree of unity never experienced before.   I repeat that we must help others to keep a sense of perspective.   There can, of course, be a backlash to these very negative and fearful feelings.   There are many occasions when one is so frustrated that the authority that decides such things, does not really think aids and adaptations are worth doing on the whole for the patient with cancer.   What is the use of giving somebody a telephone when they are going to die anyway?   My usual response is: "Well, that is the one sure thing in life. We are all going to die some time.   We could just as easily get killed to-morrow walking across a road; so, if that is the philosophy, why bother to do anything for anybody?"

        I keep coming back to the same thing - the sense of keeping things in perspective, and that malignant disease is as curable and controllable as many other conditions. Getting this message across to other social workers, both in general hospitals and the community, I see as one of the functions of the social worker in a radiotherapy unit.   The worker in a general hospital fulfils a somewhat different function.   There she provides a great deal of support to the nursing and medical staff, particularly juniors.   I think in most general hospitals the feeling, when a patient is diagnosed as having a malignant disease, is very pessimistic.   This feeling often gets over to the other patients and, whilst they do not realise what is actually the matter, there is a general feeling of depression and despondency in the ward. The social worker can do quite a lot to help this. I have spent many hours, usually in a ward kitchen, with a cup of tea, talking with nurses and young housemen about their feelings and hopes and fears. This, of course, applies in every hospital, about any condition, but malignancy is often one which brings about a feeling of helplessness and hopelessness and, when one is young and enthusiastic, one wants to cure all the world's ills, and it needs a degree of maturity to be able to accept with equanimity that there are some things of which we are not capable. Very often one has to listen to and console young people who are coming into contact with very serious illness for the very first time. The community worker often has the worst of the deal. The patients who are controlled, cured, and able to lead their own lives, rarely come into their province. They see only those who have failed to respond to treatment and need a lot of help and services which are, unfortunately, all too often unavailable. They are the ones who, often with little experience, have to support the patients and their families through a very traumatic experience. As I have said earlier, we must be prepared to support them, respect them, open up the hospital to them. More must be done, in some way, to get them involved at the early stages of the patient's illness, and to show them how to discriminate in the help and the type of help that they give; to let them see that all too often the practical problems, which are presented, are merely a displacement of the relative's feeling of complete desolation.

I have talked a lot about social work and social workers without saying much about the patient, who, after all, is the most important person of all. Obviously, to any social worker, the most important part of her work is with the patients, whether it be the lonely old lady who wants you to sit and hold her hand, or the young man fearful that coming into hospital with his terrible condition is, in some way, going to emasculate him because he can no longer be the breadwinner and provider for his family. Our acceptance of them and our willingness to help them with all their problems is surely our primary function. If we can help patients to accept the change in their way of life, a change caused by illness, we will be going a long way towards an acceptance of the disease. Two examples will suffice. If the young man who had hoped to go into heavy engineering, can be helped to

see that the change to a draughtsman's post is a feasible
and practical solution, he can believe that his life is not
over and that there is some point in studying and working;
or to help the woman who has had a mastectomy see that her
femininity has not been stolen from her and at the same time
help her husband accept that his wife has not been
"neutered," as one husband suggested to me, and that their
life as lovers can still continue.   This is all part of a
general education and a clearing away of something of the
taboo which surrounds malignancy, and social workers have a
large part to play in this, not only with our patients and
their families, but also with other colleagues and, indeed,
in our own personal relationships.

DISCUSSION

Question 1.   Currently the emphasis is upon general
social work and few workers have the opportunity to
specialise.   How do you suggest we educate Directors of
Social Services about the need to second staff to specialist
units for training and to provide further training courses
for social workers after they have had a period of general
experience?

Answer.   Unfortunately, I do not know how I can answer
this question very shortly.   I think the problem is that
it is now government policy that we take a more generic
training and that our work is more generic.   This is a
result of the Seebohm report.   If we are to go back to
specialisation, we must have new thinking.   How one
influences Directors of Social Services, I just do not know.
If somebody could tell me, I should be very grateful.

Question 2.   How can the cancer sufferer or his
relatives help other cancer sufferers to deal with their
problems?   What opportunities for this kind of social work
exist?

Answer.   I think there are many opportunities, but
just how you go about them depends on your own local area,
because, as we have already heard, many patients who have
cancer, do not, in fact, know this, so this makes forming
self-help groups not an easy proposition.   I think with
more publicity and if more patients are told what the

matter is with them, more self-help groups will be formed, and there will be much more use for counselling from people who have had the condition and have come to terms with it and are living quite normal lives again.

CANCER EDUCATION AND TRAINING - THE PUBLIC

Ian Burn

Consultant Surgeon
Charing Cross Hospital
London

In many countries of the world where there is recognised widespread poverty and enormous difficulties in travelling to and from hospitals, it is perhaps understandable that advanced malignant disease is a common occurrence. In a society such as ours, however, with all the advantages of high-powered education, sophisticated medical facilities and easy travel, it might be expected that advanced cancer would only be seen as a result of failed treatment. Such is not the case. Wards in hospitals throughout the country bear witness to this sad state of affairs, perhaps exemplified most cruelly by the appalling number of women with previously untreated advanced cancers of the breast.

Gastric cancer in this country is rarely cured and this is almost entirely due to the high proportion of patients who have advanced disease when first treated. For every 100 patients with the disease, 4 only will be alive after 10 years and cured of the disease. Although the reason for this very high mortality rate is partly due to the intrinsic nature of the disease, mostly it is due to delay in diagnosis. Symptoms caused by gastric cancer are often tolerated for a long time before medical opinion is sought, but regrettably there often is further delay by doctors before the correct diagnosis is made.

Many other malignant diseases are attended by unwarranted delay between the onset of symptoms and the start of treatment. Unlike gastric cancer, however, this delay nowadays mostly occurs between the patient first

becoming aware of symptoms and the seeking of medical advice.
A lump in the breast, cough and even mild haemoptysis, a
persistent skin lesion, bleeding per rectum and frequency of
micturation are all symptoms which occur with early malignant
disease.   They are symptoms, however, which so frequently
are rationalised by patients, even middle-aged and elderly
ones, as "mastitis," "smoker's cough," "wart," "piles and
"irritable bladder" and are tolerated for varying periods
even when the condition is worsening.   Pain, the one
symptom which usually leads to prompt action on the part of
a patient, is rarely a feature of early cancer at any site
in the body and nearly always is preceded for a long time
by other more readily tolerated symptoms, such as those
listed above.

We need to look at the reasons for this readiness to
delay seeking medical advice in the face of obvious
persistent abnormality, and why we, who are responsible for
providing information about cancer, have failed so dismally
to communicate with the public.   It is a travesty that in
a country like ours, such a high proportion of patients
present to the doctor for the first time with advanced,
inoperable, incurable cancers;   a situation which reflects
the general deep pessimism which still surrounds these
particular ailments.

Fear is frequently the cause for delay.   The woman
who delays seeking advice for a lump in the breast usually
does so because she is so frightened that it might be cancer
that she cannot bring herself to face the diagnosis.
Usually at some stage, and often after a delay of months,
she is able to overcome her fear to a point that medical
advice is sought, but by then it may be too late even to
attempt a curative procedure.   The fear is usually of the
cancer and the apparent inevitability of death rather than
the mastectomy which might be advised if the diagnosis is
made.   In general, we have failed to communicate widely
enough that the cancerous diseases can be cured if treated
early and, as we have heard from Professor Sellwood earlier,
this is paralleled by the fact that even among the caring
professions there remains widespread ignorance of the true
results of treatment.

I would like now to place some facts on record.

Fact 1.   There is no doubt that cancer is curable.
If we look at the results of treating mammary cancer, it is
clear that eventually there is a proportion of women treated,
whose survival parallels that of the normal population.
Such women correctly may be regarded as being cured because
they will live a normal life span and die from a cause other
than cancer.   It is equally clear, however, that those
patients who are cured, invariably are those who have early
disease when treated, as judged by the TNM stage of their
tumours.   Patients with T_1N_0 cancers of the breast, that is
those with tumours of less than 2 cm. and with no evidence
of spread to the regional lymph nodes and beyond, have an
almost guaranteed chance of cure with proper treatment.

Fact 2 is that no less than 20% of us in this country
are going to develop cancer, that is 1 in every 5 persons.
There is no room for complacency from any of us.   None of
us can afford to say, "It will never happen to me," because
it may very well do so.   Even if we do not fit into high-
risk groups, our chance of getting cancer is relatively
high, so we have all got an interest in this problem.

Fact 3 is that about 145,000 people each year get
cancer in the United Kingdom.   Of these cancers, 60% are
the common ones.   19,000 get cancer of the colon and
rectum, 18,000 get cancer of the breast, 16,000 get cancer
of the stomach, 15,000 get cancer of the skin and 10,000
get cancer of the female genital organs.   These are, of
course, approximate figures.   If all these patients were
diagnosed early, 80 to 85% of them would be cured and this
would represent well over the half of all the patients who
develop malignant disease in the country.   The methods of
dealing with cancer of the organs mentioned above are well
tried.   They consist of various surgical operations and
radiotherapy, singly or combined as appropriate, and they
have the ability to cure the cancers if they are diagnosed
early.

It is no exaggeration to state that, if we correctly
use the surgical and irradiation methods which we already
have available to us, and if there were no delay in diagnosis
once symptoms occur, then one half of all patients with
cancer could be cured.   There is one form of malignant
disease, however, which accounts for 20% of all cancers in
this country, for which the available treatments hold little
hope even with early diagnosis, and this, of course, is

cancer of the lung.

However soon cancer of the lung is diagnosed after
symptoms first occur, its close proximity to inaccessible
lymph node groups makes it one of the most difficult
cancers to treat effectively, either by radical surgery or
radiotherapy.   It can be eradicated almost entirely,
however, by avoiding smoking.   At present, each packet
carries on its side, in a position which few people notice,
the following ineffectual words - "Warning by Her Majesty's
Government - Smoking can Damage Your Health."   I would
like to see emblazoned across the front of every cigarette
packet the bold but nevertheless true message - "If you use
these, you are likely to die from cancer."   We have the
evidence of this in abundance, but we have failed to use
it, primarily because the intent has not been sufficiently
strong.

The concept that cancer develops in a regular fashion
from a single cell, which multiplies regularly until it
reaches a stage where it becomes clinically obvious, has
been given a lot of unjustified publicity in recent years.
It is a dangerous concept based on the flimsiest of
evidence.   It is dangerous because it implies that cancer
always exists for a long time before it becomes evident
clinically and thus the chance of dissemination having
already occurred is very high and cure, therefore, impossible.
There is no evidence that human cancers do develop from a
single cell or even a single group of cells.   All clinical
experience suggests that, far from growing in size in a
regular manner, the reverse is true.   Yet this concept of
"constant doubling time" has been used repeatedly by many
people as an argument that cancer is virtually incurable
because it can never be diagnosed early enough.   Many
clinicians who treat patients with the disease have been
influenced by this misleading philosophy.

We have failed miserably to date to communicate to the
Public the message that cancer is a curable disease and
thus create the optimism necessary to encourage people to
seek advice promptly and perhaps to participate in
programmes which are designed to detect cancer early.   As
a result of the climate created by the "constant doubling
time" theory, with its implications of inevitability, there
has been a frenzied pursuit of highly dubious so-called

systemic treatments often at the expense of proven
successful radical local surgery and radiotherapy.   The
recent excessive emphasis on systemic methods of treatment
is wrong.   There is, of course, every need to continue
exploring new avenues of treatment, but to do this at the
expense of effective, old methods, and at the expense of
pursuing the overwhelming need for early diagnosis, could
be disastrous.

Fortunately, we are becoming aware of the need for
providing proper information about cancer to the Public and
real attempts to do this are now being made.   There are a
number of independent cancer information agencies, such as
the one at Oxford, which have done and continue to do very
good work in this context.   Perhaps the new Oncological
Centres will build into their structure programmes for
helping people understand about cancer, and the British
Cancer Council must have a prominent role in co-ordinating
efforts of this type.   It is a role that the British Cancer
Council could and should fulfil very well.   But there is no
question at all that the real motivation for informing the
Public adequately about the disease must come from the
Medical Profession itself.   It must come from the doctors
who are dealing with the disease and it must reflect a
justified attitude of optimism.

I firmly believe, however, that no programme aimed at
informing the Public will be possible until the doctors
themselves reorganise the way they manage cancer.   Malignant
disease is a specialist complaint and deserves to be handled
as such.   Because of the numbers of patients involved, it
is difficult to foresee any great change soon, but we should
now be making plans for the future.

I echo Professor Sellwood's comments on the need for
the proper training of the Medical Profession and through
that will come progress in informing the General Public.
It is also important that any of the official administrative
committees that are set up to plan and to deal with public
information about cancer should contain a realistic complement
of clinicians who deal with the disease constantly, and who,
therefore, are fully familiar with all the problems involved
and the importance of the optimistic approach.   Too often
such planning committees, in matters relating to cancer, have
been overloaded with individuals, whose primary concern is
either with the academic or the financial aspects of the

problem.   For example, it is often difficult to convince
those who are not in daily contact with patients with the
disease of the overwhelming need for early diagnosis,
irrespective of the cost in financial terms.   Oncological
clinicians have a great responsibility to present their
arguments, based on practical experience, as vigorously as
possible and they should have the opportunity to do this.

Finally, I would like to make a few comments on the
role of "the media" in providing information about cancer
for the Public.   Undoubtedly the media have an increasing
responsibility to participate and television is particularly
suited to the need.   Careful planning is required to
produce programmes on various aspects of malignant disease,
which would ensure the responsible dissemination of
information to wide sections of the community.   Such
programmes probably are best organised on a regional basis,
allied to Specialist Oncological Institutes, Divisions of
Oncology or Units of Oncology, which deal with the disease.
Individual armchair philosophy by those who have nothing
more than an academic interest in the problem is to be
avoided.   If used discreetly and efficiently, television
would be of great advantage for the provision of information
on curability rates and the concept of early diagnosis, as
well as advising the Public of the facilities available for
screening for early malignant disease of the cervix and
breast, and perhaps in due course some of the more difficult
problems such as gastric cancer.

Towards the end of the 19th century, there occurred
some momentous oncological landmarks, which were entirely
concerned with surgical technique.   They included the
introduction of such revolutionary procedures as radical
mastectomy, radical gastrectomy and radical colectomy, and
they reflected considerable surgical expertise.   These
were massive operations designed because of the inadequacy
of lesser procedures, and they produced an immediate and
remarkable improvement in the results of treating cancer.

I would like to see in years to come different forms
of oncological landmarks being recorded, such landmarks
as ... "the Development of a National Screening Programme
for Cancer," ... and, "a Massive Reduction in Smoking among
the General Public," ... and, "the Introduction of a
National Register of High Risk Groups."   These are the

sort of landmarks to which we should look forward in the
future, because they will then indicate an awareness of the
Public about this particular disease.   The time has come
to adopt a new and more positive attitude about the disease.
We no longer should think in terms of cancer being a
<u>Disease which is to be Feared</u>, but rather that it is a
<u>Disease to be Cured</u>.

DISCUSSION

Question 1.   What evidence is there to demonstrate
that simply the dissemination of information leads to a
decrease in the delay in seeking medical help for suspected
cancer?

Answer.   An example of the fact that people can be
influenced by giving them information is the undoubted
success of screening for cervical cancer in California and
Western Canada.   Another example is the marked success in
Japan of screening for early gastric cancer.   In this
country, however, we do NOT have similar success stories to
report, primarily because we have not spent enough time,
energy and money on it.   The most successful commodity
that has been sold to the people of Britain in the last
twenty years is "pop" music and this has been achieved by
repetition and by a belief by those involved in the trade
in what they are doing.   We have got to bring a similar
confidence to the business of giving advice to the General
Public about cancer and the need for early diagnosis.

Question 2.   How would Mr. Burn introduce cancer
education to the schools of this country?

Answer.   This is a difficult problem because in
general we have been reluctant to bring to the notice of
children matters relating to sickness.   There has been
health care <u>of</u> children, but not a defined programme to
educate them about health.   Many children are now having
to live in families where one or other member has a cancer
and I do not think there would be any harm, for example, in
discussing certain environmental aspects of cancer.

Question 3.   Are there any psychological "trigger
points" associated with the development of cancer?   For

example, some people with cancer express deep feelings of
loss or remorse following bereavement.

Answer.   I think there are two aspects of this.   The
first is whether psychological stress can influence an
established cancerous process.   I do not think there is
any doubt that it can.   So frequently in patients with
malignant disease there does seem to be a reactivation of
apparently silent disease by psychological stress.   The
mechanism for this may well be neurochemical through centres
as yet unidentified in the region of the hypothalamus of the
brain.   The second aspect concerns the psychological effects
of developing and having to live with cancer.   I do not
think that having cancer as such, often precipitates a true
psychiatric illness, but it frequently induces marked
anxiety which in extreme cases may require the help of a
psychiatrist.

CANCER RESEARCH IN BRITAIN

M.G.P. Stoker, CBE, FRS

Director of Research
Imperial Cancer Research Fund
Lincoln's Inn Fields, London

Neither cancer nor cancer research are respectful of national boundaries, but the way research is financed and organised does vary a good deal between different countries. So I will spend a few minutes on the way cancer research is organised in Britain compared with other countries, particularly the U.S.A., where the enormous cancer programme sets an entirely new level, which sheds a light on the efforts of other countries.

CANCER RESEARCH ORGANISATIONS AND ESTABLISHMENTS

The boundaries and definitions are imprecise, but in Britain we are currently spending about £15 millions a year, or about 30p. a head. Only about a third of this is taxpayers' money, the remainder from voluntary donations to two large and several smaller private charities. The present spending in the U.S.A. is some 20 times higher, or more than 3 times higher per person, but it is nearly all government spending, the contributions from private organisations being small in relative, though not in absolute terms. In Canada, however, the system is more like our own. It is difficult to obtain figures for other western countries because private support is often confined to regions or municipalities, and used to finance research in local hospitals and laboratories.

British Government research on cancer is carried out by the Medical Research Council, indirectly by extramural grants, or directly by its own institutions and units.

135

partly through contracts in conjunction with the Department
of Health.   The Department of Health also contributes to
cancer research, but it is usually difficult to distinguish
this from patient care.   The Medical Research Council
provides the link with the international cancer efforts of
World Health Organisation and the International Agency for
Research on Cancer at Lyon, but not the International Union
Against Cancer, which is funded indirectly through private
funds.

The Cancer Research Campaign which is one of the large
charities, spends about £5 millions a year, mostly in
response to applications for support of research in
hospitals, universities and institutes throughout the
country, including some of the largest, such as the Chester
Beatty, the Paterson and the Beatson Laboratories, which
are supported jointly and in collaboration with the Medical
Research Council.

The Imperial Cancer Research Fund also spends about
£5 millions a year, if capital projects are included, but
differs from the Cancer Research Campaign in that the
research is carried out by its own staff in two large
institutes and three extramural units, all in London.   In
an important new move the Cancer Research Campaign and the
Imperial Cancer Research Fund have also endowed several
chairs in oncology in medical schools throughout the
country.

Then there are a number of important but smaller and
more specialized contributors, not least the Marie Curie
Memorial Foundation, which, as you know, devotes part of
its resources to Research at Oxted.   There is also the
more specialized Leukaemia Research Fund, and the recent
and remarkably successful Tenovus, based largely in Wales
and the South West.

Finally, the British Cancer Council, which does not
itself promote research, acts as an information and
education co-ordinator, and is the national link with the
main international voluntary organisation, the International
Union Against Cancer.

All this sounds fragmented and inefficiently
competitive, and, indeed, it was to prevent wasteful overlap

and to co-ordinate the national effort that the
Co-ordinating Committee for Cancer Research was sponsored
by the Medical Research Council, Cancer Research Campaign
and Imperial Cancer Research Fund, five years ago with a
sub-committee of the Directors of the four largest cancer
research institutes.   Apart from monitoring the main
fields of research and recommendations (though not
directions) to the sponsoring bodies, the Co-ordinating
Committee for Cancer Research has been a useful mouthpiece
on the national cancer research effort, in a way that none
of the individual research bodies could be.   When the U.K.
was invited, along with other countries, to join the
enlarged U.S. initiative against cancer, Lord Zuckerman
was asked by the Prime Minister to report on cancer
research in the U.K., and the Co-ordinating Committee for
Cancer Research was subsequently invited to respond.   In
the event, the Zuckerman Report did not judge that a
mammoth crash programme was timely in the U.K., but it did
recommend an emphasis on improved facilities for clinical
research and the research training of clinical oncologists.
The Co-ordinating Committee for Cancer Research, which had
made similar proposals, endorsed this view and made
specific recommendations to the sponsoring bodies, and the
Department of Health.   The Cancer Research Campaign and
Imperial Cancer Research Fund have themselves made an
important contribution by creation of chairs in oncology,
mostly for clinical aspects, and for other research
training schemes.   On the other hand, the delay and lack
of money for creation of the four approved cancer centres,
and the poor progress in recognition of oncology as a
speciality, has been a disappointing set-back.

SOME RECENT DEVELOPMENTS

At this bicentenary of Percivall Pott's famous paper
on cancer in chimney sweeps, let us now consider some
current research of importance.   We will note, but not
restrict ourselves to, national contributions.

To begin with we have to make a frank admission that
cancer research has so far not saved many lives, at least
in an easily quantifiable way.   Probably the most
significant group are the doctors and an unknown number of
others who would now be dead from lung cancer had it not

been for the discovery of the cancer smoking relationship concurrently by Doll and Bradford Hill in this country and by Wynder in the U.S.A. some 20 years ago.   Though less easy to quantitate, we should also remember the great contributions to prevention of industrial chemical carcinogenesis, largely associated with the Chester Beatty Research Institute over many years.

There are also, however, the patients with established cancers, for example, choriocarcinoma, whose lives have been saved in no small part through the research by Bagshaw and his colleagues, carried out here in London.   Early Hodgkin's disease and Burkitt's Lymphoma are also essentially curable, thanks to patient research in many countries and particularly the U.S.A., while the outlook for acute lymphoblastic leukaemia has improved from about 1% long time survival in 1960 to an anticipated one third in the best centres to-day.   It may be noted that the research which led to these quite remarkable advances in treatment, was not concerned with any deep understanding of fundamental biology, but mostly to new combinations of drugs originally discovered by accident, to new radiation sources developed by physicists, and to painstaking trials by clinicians.

Of particular interest at present is the research on combined immunotherapy and drug treatment of cancer.   The object is to kill as many of the cancer cells as possible with drugs, then to eliminate the remainder by maintenance courses of drugs combined with stimulation of the body's own defences against the tumour cells by vaccines to stimulate immunity.   A non-specific stimulation of immunity in leukaemia was pioneered by Mathe in Paris using BCG vaccine and is under continued trial, but a hopeful British contribution by Powles and colleagues is additional immunization by a vaccine made with irradiated leukaemia cells.   This may still not immunize specifically, but it provides a significant improvement in survival time in acute myeloid leukaemia.   It is a good example of collaboration between the major sponsoring bodies at the Royal Marsden Hospital, Sutton, supported by the Cancer Research Campaign and the Medical Research Council, and the Tumour Immunology Unit at St. Bartholomew's Hospital, one of the Imperial Cancer Research Fund's units.

The outlook in breast cancer has remained almost

unchanged for many decades despite a very large research
effort.   However, the outlook is at least beginning to
look more hopeful, not least because the surgeons and
radiotherapists are beginning to reach common ground with
physicians, endocrinologists and cell biologists, thus
allowing a much more broadly based approach to treatment
than in the past.   The progress, but not the cure, by
drugs in more advanced breast cancer has recently prompted
trials of drug treatment following surgery in early breast
cancer in Italy and the U.S.A., and more recently in the
Imperial Cancer Research Fund's Unit at Guy's Hospital.
First results after two years from the U.S.A. and Italy
look very promising, but breast cancer is a disease where
firm conclusions have to wait many years.

Even if some small progress is now in sight in breast
cancer, however, the problem of treating the established
common cancers of lung, intestine and uterus remain.   No
drugs have been developed which specifically act on cancer
cells, so all have to be used in inadequate doses because of
action on normal cells and, therefore, toxicity to the
patient through effects on the haemopoietic, immunological
and epithelial systems, all of which depend on cell
proliferation.   It is this lack of specificity which makes
us presently helpless, and encourages the long term
research which strives to identify the fundamental
differences between cancer cells and normal cells in
chemical terms.   It attracts many excellent scientists
who have identified important characteristics of tumour,
as opposed to normal cells, but so far none of them are of
a type which is leading to the design of cancer specific
drugs.

Currently, there is a great emphasis on the
alterations which are found on the surfaces of cancer cells,
and which may explain their lack of social behaviour.
Much of this promising research has been carried out in the
United Kingdom.   For example, it was Professor Ambrose at
the Chester Beatty Research Institute, who first observed
the specific effects of wheat germ extracts on tumour cells,
which led to the development by others of the plant lectins,
probably the most useful tools currently available as probes
and monitors of the cell surface.   Another quite remarkable
tool used all over the world for analysing the changes of
growth and the "muscle" mechanism of cells in division, is
a drug discovered by Dr. Stephen Carter at Imperial Chemical

Industries, Cytochalasin B.   Much more recently, with
improved and more meaningful chemical analysis of the cell
surface, Dr. Richard Hynes, working in Dr. Macpherson's
laboratory at the Imperial Cancer Research Fund, reported
a major protein constituent of the cell surface which is
profoundly altered in cancer cells, a discovery which may
have considerable ramifications.

The hope that new cancer specific antigens on the cell
surface can be used as targets after stimulation of the
immune mechanisms remains strong, and I have already
mentioned the promising immunisation programme using
leukaemic cells here in London.   It had also been hoped
that antibodies against tumour cells might be used as a
mechanism to direct cytotoxic drugs specifically to their
targets.   In fact, the antibodies and drug molecules
usually come apart before reaching the cells, but, rather
surprisingly, an adjuvant effect still exists which, though
not yet understood, could be a useful way of improving the
drug treatment.

There is another possible approach to therapy, which
comes from studies on the growth of normal and cancer cells
in culture.   Rapidly growing normal cells respond to
certain molecular hormone-like signals which start or halt
growth, while tumour cells ignore these signals.   Since
some drugs only act on dividing cells, it might be possible,
therefore, to give really large doses without fear of toxic
effects by temporarily blocking the growth of normal cells
in the immune and haemopoietic system for example, by
manipulation of the growth signalling system, and so
protecting them while the tumour cells are killed by the
cytotoxic drugs.

The recent detection in the U.S.A. of a virus from
cultured human leukaemic cells, which is closely related
to a primate cancer virus, has caused some excitement.
Here in London virologists at the Imperial Cancer Research
Fund, in a joint programme with their American colleagues,
have found how to propagate this virus, and how to test for
specific antibodies, and preliminary results suggest that
the virus may be commonly carried by human beings.
Nevertheless, the incrimination of this, or any virus, as
the primary cause of human leukaemia still remains
incomplete, and it is, anyway, obvious that leukaemia is

not infectious in the ordinary sense.   Much of the pioneer
work on viruses and natural cancer in other species has been
done in Britain, for example, the isolation of the causative
virus and first successful anticancer virus vaccine in
Marek's disease of chicken at the Poultry Research Institute,
and the virus isolation and first steps towards a vaccine
in the cat leukaemia complex in the Glasgow Veterinary
School.   The genetic evidence for endogenous tumour
viruses in nature and their activation by chemical
carcinogens was also pioneered by British virologists.
Finally, and not least, there is the discovery of the
Epstein Barr virus, a candidate for a human cancer virus if
ever there was one.

       Looking ahead at cancer treatment for the short-term,
i.e., 5 to 10 years, and following the lessons of the
successful treatment of choriocarcinoma and testicular
tumours, it now seems that the most useful research might
be directed, not to discoveries of new drugs, but to
improved use of the existing armament.   This may come in
several ways.   One is the reduction of the toxic effects
in normal tissues, for example, by normal growth inhibitors,
as I have mentioned.   The other is the development of
monitoring systems which tell the therapist the number of
tumour cells, or tumour load, before, during, and after
treatment, and then in the follow-up period.   So far, this
has only been available for choriocarcinoma, which produces
a hormone to indicate cell numbers, and hence the success
of treatment.   Probably immunological indicators of the
presence of tumour cells are likely to be of wide
application and are the subject of a good deal of effort.
Recently, a remarkable new method of monitoring the
lymphocyte population in cancer patients has been reported
from the Paterson Laboratories in Manchester, and this is
thought to be correlated with the presence of a variety of
cancers.   How it works is obscure, but will surely be
elucidated, and, anyway, despite our disquiet at the
unknown, we do not have to understand everything to make it
useful.

       I conclude with this encouraging note, but also with
a word of warning.   In that other language used by the
media, the word, "hope," especially in relation to cancer,
is almost invariably translated as "breakthrough."   I
suggest that for the sake of the public, all of whom will
either suffer from cancer, or the effects of cancer in the

family, research workers should take an oath, namely, that
they will never admit to a breakthrough.

DISCUSSION

Question 1.   Are there any proofs of cancer being a
contagious disease?   Can cancer be hereditary?

Answer.   There is no evidence that cancer itself is
a contagious disease.   Occasionally there are reports
that suggest some link between cases; for example, in
Hodgkin's disease there was a report not long ago, but it
is very doubtful, and I do not think anybody should go
about thinking that cancer patients should be kept in
isolation.   Of course, that does not mean that something
which causes cancer, might not be infectious, but
transmitted perhaps in childhood, many, many years before.

On the question of hereditary, there are some rare
forms of cancer , which are without doubt hereditary.
But the common cancers are not purely hereditary.   Many
of them have a very slight hereditary element in that, if
there is a patient with cancer in the family, there is a
slight increase in probability that another member of the
family may have cancer, either cancer in general, or the
specific type of cancer.   The effect is very small,
however, and I think should be ignored except for those
very few rare forms of cancer I mentioned.

Question 2.   May other diseases degenerate into
cancer?

Answer.   Yes, they may.   I think I should leave it
at that.

Question 3.   Is it not important that cancer research
workers should know more about cancer in humans?   How
would you suggest that facilities could be made available
to them?   How would you obtain close collaboration
between clinical and research oncologists?

Answer.   That is a difficult one to answer quickly.
We cannot expose humans to unnecessary risk by research,
so it is necessary to answer the questions with imperfect

model systems, mice, for example, or cultured cells and
such like.   The difficulty, as the questioner points out,
is to get the people who do work on mice, and obscure bits
of chemistry and so on, to appreciate the human problem –
the patient with human disease.   Research workers generally
prefer to get on with their own chosen problems where they
can answer some clear, more or less black and white questions.
However, we can organise conferences where the clinicians
with problems and the experimentalists with problems can
meet and talk about them together, and fruitful collaboration
does emerge.   But I do not think there is any quick and
easy answer.

    Question 4.   Would it be possible to isolate an
enzyme that would antagonise the dividing cell in the D.N.A?
Could a specific enzyme be developed for a particular
dividing cell?

    Answer.   Many drugs are known, which interfere with
the copying process of the D.N.A., but these affect healthy
cells as well as cancer cells.   Some are in fact used to
treat cancer, but great care is needed to avoid harmful
effects.

Part 2
CANCER — TOWARDS THE SOLUTION

Part 2

CANCER: TOWARD THE SOLUTION

ENCOURAGEMENT FROM RESEARCH ON THE CANCER OF THE INDIVIDUAL PATIENT

John R. Hobbs

Professor of Chemical Pathology
Tumour Biology Group
Westminster Hospital, London

Sir Rodney, Mr. Raven, Ladies and Gentlemen, it is a beautiful day in May and I think, rather like my illustrious namesake, I might be outside playing cricket rather than opening the innings in here. Nevertheless, here I am and much of my talk is the result of the teamwork of the Tumour Biology Group at Westminster Hospital, itself one of the evidences of advance. Instead of working in isolated groups, the surgeon in his operating theatre, the scientist in his laboratory, etc., we have a team which gets together, meets regularly and which crosses the frontiers of individual departments to achieve real co-ordination. This is one good thing that is growing in the oncological world of to-day.

There are three main themes to my title. Firstly, I do not think there is a single best treatment for any given cancer. Secondly, laboratory methods are now advancing to a degree where we really can look at the tumour of the individual patient and select the right treatment for that patient, from many treatments that are available. Thirdly, there are measurements now available from the laboratory, which can help us to monitor the progress of many cancers. One of the biggest problems with new treatments is to find out quickly how well they are doing and to-day new assays are enabling us to monitor either the products of the tumour or the damage it does to the patient in a much better way than we could even 5 years ago. Thus, I do not believe in one best treatment for all patients. I think we should look, by new methods, at the tumour of each patient to work out his or her best treatment, and finally we should

certainly develop laboratory monitoring to measure what we
are doing.

To enlarge on the first theme, let us consider current
treatments of certain cancers by cytotoxic drugs.   Such
treatments are largely being derived from massive trials,
very well-conducted and scientifically correct, in which,
for example, 100 patients with breast cancer are given one
combination of 4 cytotoxic drugs and the results compared
to those for 100 patients given a different combination, to
prove statistically that the quadruple regime is 10 per cent
better.   We finish with the single best treatment for all
patients with recurrent breast cancer.   While this may be
the most economic way to go ahead, we already know that,
when such patients relapse from cytotoxic treatment, the
incidence of those who might now respond to hormone ablation,
is reduced from 53 per cent to 29 per cent. (1)   So, half
such patients may have been deprived of the chance of
responding to hormone therapy by first treating them with
cytotoxic drugs.   While for a statistical group the latter
was the best single treatment, yet for a given patient whose
tumour has been carefully tested, it might be possible to
have chosen a better treatment.

At the Westminster Hospital, when our histopathologist
has made his diagnosis of breast cancer on the tumour
biopsy, a portion from the growing edge is sent to our Dame
Barbara Hepworth Laboratory for special studies.   Small
pieces are placed in a dish of tissue culture medium and to
different dishes are added different known hormones. (1)
Known cytotoxic drugs (2) can also be added.   This is done
to find out which, if any, hormones encourage the tumour
and we can also study which substances can inhibit tumour
growth.

Where the added hormone promotes the tumour we can see
an increase in enzyme activity as compared to controls
without the added hormones in the cultured cancer cells,
i.e., the hormone induces synthesis of enzyme.   Where
inhibition results we can see a decrease, but, if there is
no obvious inhibition or promotion, we consider the cancer
is independent in vitro of the added substances.

For the last 100 years surgeons have been taking their
biopsies and dropping them into formalin and I think to-day

this is the biggest disservice they can do to the patient
with breast cancer.   While the tissue is still alive, it
can be used to test, not only for hormone dependence, but
also for cytotoxic sensitivity and immunological parameters.
It can also be stored by controlled freezing in liquid
nitrogen, and our tumour bank now contains over 500 various
cancers which help us in other attempts to design treatment
should a given patient return with a recurrence.

Table 1.   Laboratory culture results for 550 breast cancer
            patients.

Pattern No.

1	47% Independent	
	53% Dependent	
2	Prolactin/Growth Hormone (GH)	16%
3	Prolactin/GH or Oestrogen	12%
4	Prolactin/GH or Androgen	11%
5	Prolactin/GH or Oestrogen or Androgen	1%
6	Androgen only	5%
7	Oestrogen only	8%
	In pregnancy	
8	2 patients - Prolactin/GH or Human Placental Lactogen	

Table 1 shows the results from 550 breast cancers.
About half the tumours are classed as independent.   These
are tumours which we believe have dedifferentiated (grown
away) from the natural breast epithelium which is hormone
responsive.   They can now thrive without hormones and they
will not respond, we know now, to any attempt at hormone
ablation.   But the other half of breast cancers appear to
be dependent and you will see that they can show seven
different patterns of dependence.   Prolactin and growth
hormone dependence almost always occur together.   Oestrogen
or androgen dependence can occur alone or with dependence on
other hormones.   A given tumour showing multiple dependences
can be promoted by any one of the hormones.

In Table 1 there are eight different kinds of breast

cancer in terms of their hormone profile, so that right away
there is obviously no single treatment which can counter all
of these patterns.   For pattern 2 you can only use
hypophysectomy.   For pattern 6 adrenalectomy can be used.
For pattern 7 you might use oophorectomy.   If you must have
a single best treatment for all, it would mean taking out
nearly every endocrine organ in the body.   By studying the
tumour of the individual patient we try to select the
treatment most likely to help her.

        Table 1 could be very relevant to the latest breast
cancer trials in Europe, (3) where the use of high dose
oestrogen produced regression in 14 per cent of patients,
and an anti-oestrogen produced regressions in 31 per cent.
The conclusion was that, although the response rate to the
anti-oestrogen seemed best, its side effects were too
frequent to recommend its use.   The assumption was made that
the two treatments affected the same sub-group of patients
with recurrent breast cancer.   We would argue that the 14
per cent of patients that responded to high oestrogen were
the androgen-dependent tumours and that the 31 per cent of
patients who responded to the anti-oestrogen were the
oestrogen-dependent tumours.   Had they done a crossover
study in their trial, it is possible there could have been a
45 per cent response rate overall.   They did not report any
tests at all to tell you what kind of tumour might have
responded.   This was just another one of those "blunderbuss"
trials.

        Now the technique we have used does show that in the
pre-menopausal woman there is more dependence on prolactin
57% and oestrogen 32% and in the post-menopausal more
dependence on androgen 26%.

        The technique in culture is a tricky one and cannot
readily be set up in every hospital in Great Britain.   We
have, therefore, developed a new approach in the last year.
Prolactin, growth hormone and human placental lactogen seem
to act by attaching themselves to receptors on the cell
membrane.   Thus, for example, prolactin is allowed to bind
to the cell membrane in thin sections of breast cancer and
then free prolactin is washed away.   A rabbit antibody to
the prolactin is then allowed to bind and the excess then
washed away.   Bridge antibodies are now allowed to bind to
the first rabbit antibodies.   As they are added in excess,
free sites are available to bind to further rabbit antibodies

against an enzyme peroxidase.   In this way several
peroxidase molecules are bridged to where the prolactin
originally bound.   Thousands of molecules of peroxidase
substrate can now be acted on by the bridged peroxidase to
develop a brown colour where the prolactin bound.   This new
system is about 1,000 - 10,000 times more sensitive than the
older fluorescent antibody methods.   It can work within
three hours and we believe can actually detect the presence
or absence of prolactin receptors on the membranes of the
cancer cells.   There is a 92 per cent correlation (4) with
our culture results.   Thus, two independent methods, added
hormone promoting the culture, or the detection of the
receptors on the surfaces of the cells agree in selecting
which tumours might be prolactin-dependent.   The latter
method could become more widely used.

Of the patients tested only 89 have been available for
assessment after receiving only anti-hormonal treatments and
the laboratory predictions have been wrong in 17 per cent and
correct in 83 per cent.   Thus, when an individual patient
presents with a recurrence of breast cancer, laboratory
studies of the tumour biopsy can help to select treatment.
When hormone dependence is suggested, a trial of anti-
hormonal treatment is the first choice because prior use of
radiotherapy or cytotoxic drugs can halve the chances of a
subsequent hormonal response.   This same type of approach
can also be explored for carcinoma of the prostate, and
carcinoma of the body of the uterus, for preliminary studies
indicate that about half of these cancers are also hormone
dependent.

The above evidence supports, I hope, my contention that
there is no one best treatment for women with recurrent
breast cancer, and this concept is probably true for certain
other cancers, such as, prostatic.   Instead we should move
to the wider use of laboratory help with the tumour biopsies
to try and select the best treatment for an individual
patient at that particular time.

Turning now to my third theme, the monitoring of cancer,
the advances here derive from the increasing number of
products of tumours, that can be measured in serum or urine
samples to give an earlier indication of what is happening.

The value of such measurements was clearly established

during the myeloma trials of a Medical Research Council Working Party. These began in 1964, when melphalan and similar drugs had been available for some 5 years. Despite this, the 2-year survival of patients from a diagnosis of myelomatosis was only 8 per cent. With the 98 per cent reliable monitoring achieved (5) by careful measurements of myeloma protein products, better management followed and now with the same drugs the 2-year survival of patients is 56 per cent, the 5-year close to 30 per cent and the 10-year survival at 12 per cent, unheard of 20 years ago.

I credit most of this to the fact that we now know what we are doing because we are measuring what is happening to the tumours. It has been possible to detect them at a size of only 3-30 g., e.g., from a small pea to about a walnut.

Following on that teamwork has been the even more rewarding work by Professor Bagshawe's group (6) in this country. Measuring human chorionic gonadotrophin, a product of choriocarcinoma, they have been able to institute chemotherapy when the tumour has been only "pea-size" and thus prevent completely the horrific growths I saw as a medical student in 1954, when a woman could die from this disease in less than one year after the removal of a hydatidiform mole. About half of all choriocarcinomas occurred in this way, and with monitoring that half are now cured.

Another tumour marker, alpha-feto protein is being used to monitor malignant hepatoma and hepatoblastoma and teratoma. (7) In children in France, Uriel (8) has on 4 occasions found alpha-fetoprotein still persisting in the blood despite an operation to remove the hepatoblastoma. He has, therefore, performed a second operation to remove more of the liver, including the last bit of tumour, and has abolished the alpha-fetoprotein level. Thus 4 children are alive and well instead of dying from residual tumour which would have killed all of them within two years. This is another less frequent, but very dramatic, success showing how monitoring can be used to indicate "second-look" surgery.

We have also the history of carcino-embryonic antigen, where since 1965 all the effort concentrated on diagnosis, and measurements eventually proved (9) to be not much better than the current techniques available. This is because many regenerative states also produce detectable levels, (i.e., the false positive rate would be too high if set at a low level,) so that a good difference in level is only found when most tumours have passed the size of a walnut.   When, however, in recent years CEA has been used to monitor the progress of the cancer, it can give an early indication of relapse.   For example, in a patient with breast cancer, her serum showed a measurable level of C.E.A. before the first operation, which reduced the level to the normal range. Ten months later the serum level was found to be rising. Yet it was not until 20 months later that the actual metastases became clinically evident.   So, it is possible to obtain a 10-month "lead time" on the recurrence of the tumour.   That can enable the recurrent tumour to be detected at a small size, instead of waiting until obvious metastases or recurrence occur.

Another assay evaluated in breast cancer is that for casein, a protein of normal breast milk.   A combination of casein and C.E.A. assays in Franchimont's laboratory (10) in Liege, seems capable of detecting 90 per cent of recurrences occurring in patients with breast cancer.

Other tumour markers are also under evaluation for many cancers and a current list is given in Table 2.   With such measurements we can, with up to 90 per cent confidence, treat some recurrent tumours.   In general when the level is reduced the treatment is being successful and where treatment fails the level rises.   I consider that this is a tremendous advance, although, as is usual in clinical medicine, it is not foolproof.   Some tumours continue to grow but lose their markers, so the measurements are misleading, as in 2 per cent of myelomatosis and perhaps 10 per cent of teratomas.   Such monitoring also enables earlier assessments of therapeutic trials.   Furthermore, they can be applied to guide the treatment of the individual patient.   It will also be possible to screen certain high-risk cancer groups.   Some of these tumour markers correlate with inhibition of the patient's ability to reject foreign cells; thus, with metastatic melanomatosis we find measurable levels of a melanoma marker. (11)   While this is high in the plasma of the patient, that plasma can inhibit the mixed lymphocyte reaction, a test of the capacity of T-lymphocytes to reject foreign cells.   When the level is lowered by plasma exchange treatment (12) the inhibitory capacity is lost.

With such measurements we are trying to select those patients who might benefit from such plasma exchange so that they might be able to reject their own tumour. Finally, a rather elegant use, some of the antibodies made against these tumour markers will home back on the tumours, for some of the markers are actually produced on the membranes of the tumour cells. Thus, a child had a neuroblastoma removed, and, from the live tumour, culture lines were established. Irradiated tumour cells were used to raise antibodies, and these were harvested and purified to be tumour-specific (not reacting with the normal tissues of the child.) To the purified antibodies was attached a cytotoxic drug, chlorambucil, and they were then given intravenously to the child, who had a bone marrow extensively invaded by tumour cells. That the antibodies had "homed" on these tumour cells was proven in two ways: firstly, the child had a dramatic remission, maintained for 9 months with a marked reduction of tumour cells in the bone marrow; secondly, special methods localised both the antibodies and the chlorambucil on the membranes of tumour cells identified in a bone marrow aspirate. (See Fig. 1) The already possible value of monitoring tumour markers is summarised in Table 3.

I think the era has come when we must save the tumour material removed from patients; it must not all go into formalin. Studies, such as discussed here, could not have been made if the tumour cells had not been grown in culture. In such new ways, tumours can be studied to find out whether or not they are hormone-dependent, or are susceptible to a cytotoxic drug, or carry a tumour marker. In such ways, progress can be made to design the treatment for the individual patient based on the studies of their own tumour.

Table 2.   Tumour markers being applied to the monitoring of human cancers.

I.   Established and in regular use:

1. Paraproteins in B-lymphocyte neoplasms: Waldenstrom; Hobbs; Salmon

2. Alpha-feto-protein (AFP) in hepato-carcinoma and teratoma: Abelev; Tatarinov; Kohn; Hirai; Uriel

3. Carcinoembryonic antigen (CEA) in gut and epithelial cancers:
Gold; Burtin

4. Chorionic gonadotrophin (HCG) in hydatidiform mole and choriocarcinoma:
Bagshawe

II. Becoming established:

1. Kappa-casein for breast, stomach and lung:
Franchimont

2. Melanoma antigen:
Bennett & Cooke; Carrel

III. Promising:

1. Neuroblastoma antigen:
Bennett & Cooke

2. Gamma-feto-protein:
Old

3. Beta-feto-protein:
Fritsche & Mach

4. Hypernephroma antigen:
Talberg; Retsas & Hobbs; Gruenwald

5. Oncofetal pancreatic antigen:
Banwo, Versey & Hobbs; Gelder & Hunter

6. Pregnancy-associated macroglobulin (PAM):
Stimson

7. Mammal carcinoantigen (MCA):
Schafer; Nielsen

8. Bronchial tumour associated antigen:
Rogers

9. Ectopic hormones:
Landon

IV. Not recommended as too non-specific:

1. Fetal isoferritin (alpha-2-H):
Von Kleist; Alpert

2. Neoplastic cross-reacting antigen (NCA):
Burtin

      3. Fetal sulphoglycoprotein antigen (FSA):
         Hakkinen

      4. Tissue polypeptide antigen (TPA):
         Bjorklund

V.   Not-tumour specific but of general use:

      1. Prostatic acid phosphatase:
         Huggins

      2. Total hydroxyproline (OHP) urinary output
         or OHP/creatinine ratio for bony metastases:
         Ziff; Guzzo; Powles

      3. Polyamine ratios to monitor the growth
         versus necrosis:
         Salmon

      4. Numerous enzymes and isoenzymes, but usually
         for only a minority of a given cancer:
         Fishman

Table 3. Value of tumour markers.

      1. Of limited value in primary diagnosis due to
         lack of sensitivity (usually $>10^9$ cells)
         and/or specificity (false positive rate.)

      2. Allow earlier assessments of therapeutic trials.

      3. Detection of residual tumour can initiate
         second-look surgery/post primary treatments.

      4. Enable earlier treatment of recurrences.

      5. To screen high-risk groups (1° or 2°).

      6. Where correlation occurs with 'blocking' of
         the patient's immune response, they can guide
         immunotherapy.

      7. Can sometimes be the target for passive
         immunotherapy.

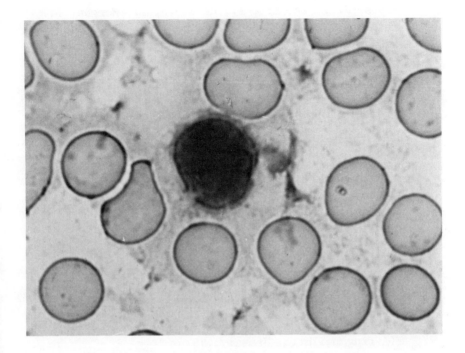

Figure 1.   In the centre is a neuroblastoma tumour cell
             in the bone marrow taken from the patient.
             The dark rim around the nucleus is due to
             peroxidase substrate precipitated where the
             chlorambucil-gammaglobulin has become fixed
             to the nuclear membrane.   The ordinary
             limiting cell membrane can be seen outside
             this.   This unusual localisation was seen
             in all the neuroblastoma cells found in the
             bone marrow and did not occur in any of the
             other nucleated cells.

REFERENCES

1. Hobbs, J.R., Barrett, A., de Souza, I., Morgan, L.,
   Raggat, P. and Salih, H. (1975) Host Defense
   Against Cancer and its Potentiation. Ed.D.Mizuno,
   Univ. Tokyo Press, p. 435.

2. Holmes, H.L. and Little, J.M. (1974) Lancet ii, 985.

3. Heuson, J.C. et al. (1975) Hormones and Breast Cancer.
   Ed. M. Namer and C.M. Lalanne, p. 247.   Paris,
   Inserm, 1975.

4. De Souza, I., Salih, H., Hobbs, J.R. and Robyn, C.
   (1976) Protides Biol. Fluids 24, in press.

5. Hobbs, J.R. (1969) Br. J. Haemat. 16, 607.

6. Leader (1974) Brit. Med. J. 3, 543.

7. Kohn, J. and Weaver, P. (1974) Lancet ii, 334.

8. Uriel, Y., Nechaud, B., Ann. Inst. Pasteur (1972)
   122, 829.

9. FDA Drug Bulletin, January, 1974.

10. Hendrick, J.C. and Franchimont, P. (1974) Europ. J.
    Cancer 10, 725.

11. Bennett, C., Cooke, K.B. and Geck, P. (1976) Protides
    Biol. Fluids 24 in press.

12. Oon, C.J. and Hobbs, J.R. (1975) Clin. Exp. Immunol.
    20, 1.

DISCUSSION

Question 1.   In what ways does Professor Hobbs consider
that human cancer research can be expanded?

Answer.   To-day there is now growing a capacity to move
across into human systems;   certainly by cell cultures, and
I think some of the advances in cancer research will be
coming from studies on the human tumours themselves.   There

are increasing numbers of human cell lines which are long-
lasting and stable in repeated culture.   There is also more
work being done on short-term cultures of tumours that come
from patients, such as, those we discussed this morning.
These have the advantage that they are more representative
of the varieties of human cancer we have to treat.   After
all, thousands of experiments on one inbred strain of rats,
or even on one long-term human cell line usually only each
represent a single type of tumour.   We need to find out
more about the variations shown by the individual patients.

     Question 2.   I have a critical question for Professor
Hobbs.   I am not sure whether it is a question about his
success or about other people's failure but here it is.
Professor Hobbs, your technique for assessing hormone
sensitivity of breast tumours has been repeated by numerous
workers up and down the country and all have failed to
confirm your results.   Please comment.

     Answer.   I am pleased to comment on this because it is
true that our technique is difficult and I think we must
admit this right away, but I would not say it was numerous
workers.   There were two groups in Britain, who tried to
set up our method, neither of whom came to see us first.
Others would consider an early visit to the original
laboratory as of prime importance.   As eventually published,
their methods were not exactly the same as ours.   Reasons
why we think they failed are in our letter (Lancet (1976)
ii, 1034.)   On the other side, the Charing Cross Group and
our Group can make the method work.   We are using a concept
that adding the hormone makes a dependent tumour synthesise
more of an enzyme.   Well, now, that concept, which we put
forward four years ago, has been successfully applied by at
least nine different groups (references available) around
the world, measuring various products in response to the
added hormones.   Our concept is confirmed;   our methodology
is difficult, and I hope it will be simplified in the future.

     Question 3.   What specific contributions to human cancer
treatment have been made by laboratory cancer research on
animals?

     Answer.   There is an enormous number of treatments,
which have their origin in good animal research, and I think
perhaps the two big fields are irradiation therapy and
chemotherapy.   A large amount of the fractional dosage, and

the right way to give irradiation and the right intervals, have all been worked out in experimental animal models. For this kind of work it is essential to have an intact animal with a circulation and the variation in oxygenation that is going to be encountered in patients. In the area of cytotoxic drugs, we now know, of course, that a large number of these have been developed and tested out on whole animals to show the effects on all kinds of tissues in the intact state before they have been given to human beings, and I would hate to be without the experimental animals for these purposes. I would like to add, however, that, wherever possible, we ourselves do use tissue cultures of human tumours, etc., as I have illustrated in my talk.

Question 4. What are the growing points of chemical pathology in relation to human cancer?

Answer. Chemical pathology has spent too much of its time in the past fifteen years in developing automation for its own sake. However, in the field of cancer the ability to detect and measure tumour markers in samples from patients is going to be a major growing area in the next ten years. I would predict most clinical value will be in the follow-up of patients with known cancers. Frankly, we cannot afford screening of the normal population, which incidentally has yet to be shown to be cost-effective. (See Hobbs, J.R.(1974) Lancet ii, 1305.) However, in follow-up, current services would need much less extra money to improve, e.g., total urinary hydroxyproline in a chemical pathology department is as good as the Scintiscan for bone metastases and costs about one-fiftieth of it. Tables 2 and 3 in my paper list the areas in which chemical pathologists will be able to help oncologists institute earlier and better controlled treatments.

Question 5. Reference has been made to the risk of endometrial tumour with hormone replacement therapy. What are your views?

Answer. Really, this is more for the expert knowledge of Dr. F. Roe, but I can comment on oestrogens. It is well established, since they were first discovered, that excess oestrogens per se can induce cancers, and perhaps the most dramatic examples are in men given high doses for metastatic carcinoma of the prostate when they develop carcinoma of the breast. I personally have encountered five such cancers,

as against only two spontaneous male breast cancers over the
same period.   The evidence suggests synthetic oestrogens may
be more dangerous (B.M.J. 1976, 2, 791.)   Those used in
various contraceptive pills are also under scrutiny.
(B.M.J. 1976, 1, 545;   Lancet 1976, i, 843.)   Nevertheless,
in replacement dosage in menopausal women such risks may be
very small and should be judged against the benefits:
quite apart from feeling better and not committing suicide
during a depressive phase, such patients do experience far
fewer deaths from fractured neck of the femur.   The papers
so far published have not produced proper credit and balance
sheets allowing for all sides, so I would rather keep an open
mind at present, and hand over to Dr. Roe.

    Dr. F. Roe.   Perhaps I may just add a view to that.
I think hormones should be likened to very sharp chisels.
They are instruments with which you can do very fine work
and you can also do a great deal of harm.   I think it is,
therefore, very important, wherever hormones are given in
therapy, to monitor what one is doing in relation to cancer.
Hormones may cause cancer.   They may greatly benefit the
patient with cancer.   I think another point is, where one
uses this glib term, hormone replacement therapy, I think it
is very important to make sure that replacement is replacement
and is not an excessive dose to somebody who does not, in
fact, need it.

    Question 6.   (1) What are the results in your
department of using "inappropriate" therapy, (e.g., endocrine
therapy for tumours without in vitro hormone dependence?)

            (2) What criteria of response are you
using when claiming 80% success for 'individualised' therapy
for advanced breast cancer cases?

    Answer.   (1) (a) The effects first of all of giving
hormones to patients with tumours independent in vitro.
When we first began this about 5 years ago, the surgeons
were free to do what they wished.   As a result, there were
5 hypophysectomies;   all failed to induce any form of
improvement.   There were also about 60 patients who had some
kind of anti-hormonal therapy, and among these the response
rate was about 5%.   The occasional patient responded to
Durabolin or Tamoxifen when we had not found any hormone
dependence in culture.   Overall, where we find that the
tumour of a patient is independent in vitro by our method,

the chances of getting a response are as small as those
reported for oestrogen-receptor negative patients in America.

(1) (b) There is another form of 'inappropriate'
therapy: the giving of hormones to a tumour showing in vitro
dependence.   For the only two patients with oestrogen-
dependent tumours given oestrogen, and for the only two
patients with androgen-dependent tumours given androgen, we
recorded alarming increases in the rate of tumour growth in
all patients.   Since then our colleagues have taken more
notice of the in vitro results, and there have been no more
patients to assess.

(2) The criteria for response we adopt are
similar to those recommended by the British Cancer Group.
We like to see 50% reduction in measureable tumour, or in a
measureable parameter, such as, hydroxyproline excretion,
preferably maintained for six months.   However, we have
reduced this to three months to get an earlier assessment
because we usually find that it is maintained in most
patients for the six months.   If it does not show within
six weeks, we are prepared to abandon the anti-hormonal
measures and pass the patient on for other forms of treatment.
For our patients, we are not just trying to remove or oppose
the hormone to which the tumour shows in vitro response, we
are also checking that it is being removed by plasma hormone
assays or is opposed in vitro.   Furthermore, for the
patients included in our reports, the anti-hormonal therapy
had to be the only treatment.   It is known that local
radiotherapy can have remote effects on other metastases.
That is why we are talking about small numbers of patients:
only 22 hypophysectomies, 11 oophorectomies, etc., and we
must admit that we would like to increase these numbers.
We can at least feel sure that we are doing no worse than
those assessing oestrogen receptors.

CANCER - NEW HOPE FOR YOUNG AND OLD

Ronald W. Raven, O.B.E., O.St.J., T.D.

Royal Marsden Hospital and Institute of Cancer
Research, Royal Cancer Hospital
London

The most important cancer discovery during the last
forty years is that not only do chemicals cause cancer,
they also cure cancer.   The causation and cure of cancer
have been sought by clinicians and scientists for centuries.
Chemical carcinogenesis and chemotherapy are important
advances towards the solution and provide good reason of
giving new hope for young and old.   This advance is the
result of team work in many clinics and laboratories all
over the world, following the fundamental research work of
Kennaway, Haddow and colleagues at the Institute of Cancer
Research, Royal Cancer Hospital, London.   No spectacular
breakthrough is, therefore, claimed to-day, neither do I
expect this to happen in the future.   The same patient team
work must continue in the years ahead until we reach the
goal.   Nevertheless, we can say to-day that many cancers,
even the most dangerous, are preventable and curable.

Cancer now has a new look.   This should be seen
clearly by the public who can be encouraged by this new
hope.   I would like the word, cancer, abolished altogether,
for it has no scientific meaning and causes people to have
tremendous apprehension of suffering and death.   There is
no need for this and I advocate the substitution of the term,
oncological diseases, as being logical and accurate.   Under
this heading are many different diseases, preventable and
curable, requiring various methods of diagnosis and treatment.
We speak of dermatological and gynaecological diseases, why
not oncological diseases which are masterminded by the
multidisciplinary science of oncology.   I believe this
particular change would be profoundly beneficial for us all.

CURATIVE TREATMENT

Although prevention is better than curing diseases, I
will deal first with curative treatment, for this has always
gripped the imagination more strongly, and, like our
ancestors two thousand years ago, we still look for miracles
to-day.

All diseases, including oncological diseases, are best
treated before obtaining a firm hold on the patient.   An
accurate early diagnosis gives the best chance for a cure,
and this can be achieved, even before any symptoms or a
tumour appear, with our modern screening techniques.   These
include cytological, radiological and biochemical methods,
and I mention particularly the exciting new system of
computerized tomography by the EMI scanner.   We are using
this for the diagnosis of brain and skull tumours, and
doubtless this will soon be used for tumours in other parts
of the body.

Spectacular advances have been made in methods of
curative treatment, and surgery has a brilliant record for
saving countless lives.   Large numbers have been cured by
radiotherapy, which has developed remarkably since Marie and
Pierre Curie discovered radioactivity, and how much they
would have rejoiced with us to-day in seeing the establishment
of another major form of treatment with various chemicals,
including hormones.

Clinicians, surgeons, physicians and radiotherapists
now see clearly that the results of their particular
treatment can be improved greatly by combinations of methods.
Pre- and post-operative radiotherapy has been used with
beneficial effects, and now we all realise the present and
potential value of the judicious use of different chemicals,
either alone, or in combination with surgery.   We have
evidence that chemicals will sensitize tumours for more
effective radiotherapy, and make others smaller for surgical
removal.   Chemicals are also used to kill malignant cells
in the blood stream, thereby preventing metastases.   This
is a good beginning, for we realise the need for chemicals
with a greater selective disease effect, without any
deleterious action on normal tissues.   They should also be
easy to administer to patients for long periods to maintain
them in good health.   Chemicals revolutionized the treatment
of infectious diseases and the particular bacteria are typed

for the appropriate antibiotic.   We are searching for new
chemicals for leukaemias and tumours, and already have
devised a system for typing breast carcinoma cells for the
appropriate chemical treatment.   In the 1930's I was one
of the first to use a synthetic chemical for a patient with
a hopeless bladder carcinoma, which regressed remarkably,
but now we have a wide range from which to choose to suit
particular patients in every age group.

THE CARE OF CHILDREN

Some of the most dangerous oncological diseases affect
children.   They are the second cause of total mortality in
the young, and a big effort is being made by researchers and
clinicians to halt this loss of life.   For instance,
prospective joint research by the Marie Curie Memorial
Foundation and Oxford University is concerned with
transplacental carcinogenesis, virus infections and
environmental hazards in pregnant women to reduce the
incidence in children.

Leukaemia is the commonest of these diseases under 15
years, followed by tumours of the central nervous system and
then by various sarcomas, including the dangerous
neuroblastoma, nephroblastoma and rhabdomyosarcoma.   The
future for them all is brightening considerably.

Approximately fifteen per cent of children with acute
lymphoblastic leukaemia treated with combinations of
chemicals are enjoying good quality life five and more years
later.   We seek constantly better ways to use chemicals for
these patients.   A good example is intrathecal injections
to destroy leukaemic cells in the central nervous system,
when meningeal symptoms are dramatically controlled.

Brain tumours, the commonest solid tumours in children,
cause distressing paralyses and other symptoms.   Following
accurate information about their size and position from the
EMI scanner and concerning their nature from surgical biopsy,
definitive treatment by surgery and radiotherapy, alone or
combined, is carried out.   This treatment now cures an
appreciable number of children, who return to normal life.

Other tumours in the head and neck region causing

distressing deformities are the result of rhabdomyosarcoma
and Burkitt's lymphoma.   The former regresses dramatically
with combined radiotherapy and chemotherapy, if it cannot
be removed, and the latter may melt away after the initial
dose of chemotherapy.

A cure rate of eighty five per cent can be achieved
with the serious retinoblastoma.   With combined surgery,
radiotherapy and chemotherapy, there is a cure rate of
eighty per cent of children with the dangerous Wilm's tumour
(nephroblastoma).   I could speak of other tumours responsive
to combined treatment but must mention thyroid carcinoma
which metastasizes to the cervical lymph nodes and lungs.
Here surgical removal of the thyroid gland with the regional
lymph nodes followed by external radiotherapy to the neck
and radioiodine treatment to the lungs can cure the patient.

Finally, chemotherapy brings new hope to children with
an osteosarcoma of a long bone, for they are now living
without evidence of disease forty months after an amputation
and continuing treatment with chemicals.   The next advance
is to save the limbs of these children, as well as their
lives, which is a distinct possibility.   We are considering
the practicality of removing the affected bone, as the femur
or humerus, and inserting a metal replacement to restore
function of the limb.   I feel we can all agree to-day there
are many good reasons for this brighter hope for the young.

THE CARE OF ADULTS

Oncological diseases occur during every period of adult
life, although their variety and behaviour are different in
various age groups.   The results of surgery and radiotherapy,
alone or combined, exemplified by the restoration of
individual patients to normal life, or by the newly published
fifteen year survival rates by the Registrar-General for the
United Kingdom, are extremely encouraging.   It can be
predicted with confidence that these results will become
much better with the increasing use of chemicals, especially
as adjuvant treatment with surgery and radiotherapy.   I
will consider briefly some of these important developments.

Lymphomas.   This is a large group of tumours, including
Hodgkin's disease, which occur in children and adults, where
treatment used to be palliative only, without any thought of

cure, and the patients died quickly.   This attitude has
changed completely, especially in Hodgkin's disease, where
surgery, radiotherapy and chemotherapy are always used,
either singly or in combination.   The most beneficial
results are obtained, for a complete remission from the
disease can be achieved in the great majority of patients,
which may be for so long that a permanent cure can be
visualized for some.

Carcinomas of the Alimentary Tract.   These are common
and serious, but their treatment with combined methods is
giving very encouraging results.   Large, inoperable
carcinomas in the thoracic oesophagus regress with combined
radiotherapy and chemotherapy to restore normal deglutition.
We have learned it is important first to establish a
gastrostomy under local anaesthesia to maintain the patient's
nutritional state at its optimum throughout the period of six
weeks' treatment.

Carcinoma of the stomach is usually advanced when
patients are first seen for surgical treatment;   so the
prognosis is grave.   It is now most significant to find that
this disease will respond favourably to chemicals, including
5-Fluorouracil and Methotrexate, and perhaps others too.
When a gastric carcinoma is too advanced for removal,
combined radiotherapy and chemotherapy can be most beneficial
in causing tumour regression.   The administration of
chemicals following gastrectomy may also control residual
disease which cannot be removed.

Combined treatment has developed for carcinoma of the
colon and rectum.   Post-operative chemotherapy with
5-Fluorouracil or quadruple therapy is given for residual,
recurrent or metastatic disease, either alone or combined
with radiotherapy.

Breast carcinoma is the commonest malignant tumour in
women, causing us considerable concern because of its
dangerous and unpredictable nature.   Several treatments are
given for different varieties and stages of this disease.
A most dramatic method is the manipulation of hormone control
mechanisms by oophorectomy, adrenalectomy, hypophysectomy,
or the administration of synthetic hormones, which can cause
the carcinoma to heal for many years and give lives of good
quality to patients with metastatic disease.   Using scanning

techniques we find that about twenty per cent of patients
have systemic breast carcinoma when first seen.   Consequently
systemic treatment is essential for them, which is now
provided by chemicals.   It has been proved already that a
high remission rate is achieved in these patients.   Following
these encouraging results with systemic disease, chemicals
are now given to patients undergoing mastectomy, who have
metastatic axillary lymph nodes.   When further proof of the
value of adjuvant chemotherapy is available from controlled
clinical trials, chemicals will likely be used in combination
with surgery for patients with negative axillary nodes.

The present availability of three dimensional therapy
for the oncological diseases is extremely encouraging.   Its
assessment by controlled clinical trials is necessary so
that further advances are made.   More effective, specific
and safer chemicals are needed, with scientific explanations
of their cellular actions.   All this work requires team
work by clinicians and researchers;   the clinic and the
laboratory are one.

In addition to adults in general, I want to give a
word of encouragement and hope to patients who are elderly,
because octogenarians and older people unfortunately develop
these diseases, although less commonly than those in younger
age groups.   It is the patient's biological age, rather
than the calendar age, that matters.   The old are assessed
like the younger patients to judge whether they are fit
enough to undergo the appropriate treatment.   I find that
many octogenarians undergo an operation without difficulty,
which may relieve them of distressing symptoms from the
tumour.   Other patients benefit from radiotherapy or
chemotherapy, and this may be given as visiting patients.
They all need supportive treatment, especially for their
nutrition.   When home nursing is necessary, this can be
provided by the Foundation's Day and Night Nursing Service.

PREVENTIVE TREATMENT

Preventive medicine has never attracted the interest
and effort it undoubtedly merits, possibly because its
results are not visible, or so dramatic, as those of
curative medicine.   For the control of oncological diseases
prevention is our great hope, because about seventy per cent

can be prevented if people took the right action.
Epidemiological research has revealed a large number which
are caused by factors in our environment, by our habits and
customs.   Laboratory research has made spectacular
discoveries concerning the carcinogenic action of chemicals
on our organs and tissues.   The grave risk from asbestos
exposure was publicized recently, although for many years
we have recognized the association of malignant tumours of
the lung, pleura, peritoneum, stomach, large bowel and
other organs with asbestos.   All this means we can protect
ourselves in different ways from these serious risks and
remain healthy for our normal life span.   Prevention,
therefore, gives new hope to everyone, young and old,
provided we undertake our responsibilities seriously to
keep fit.

Responsibility in Pregnancy

A healthy child at birth depends upon its normal
development in utero and the exclusion of any factor that
affects it adversely.   Consequently the responsibilities
of the pregnant woman are emphasized to eliminate anything
which is deleterious to the foetal tissues.   For example,
we know that injurious chemicals, including nicotine, can
pass through the placenta to reach the foetus, causing
damage to these developing organs and tissues in their most
vulnerable state.   Furthermore, chemical carcinogens
administered to pregnant animals can produce tumours in
their offspring.   Smoking tobacco during pregnancy can
cause babies to be underweight, and perhaps other
abnormalities too.   There are reports of an increased risk
of carcinoma of the vagina in the daughters of women who
were treated with diethylstilboestrol during the relevant
pregnancies.

It is strongly advised that pregnant women should not
smoke tobacco and not take chemicals, either drugs or
hormones, unless prescribed by doctors.   Constant vigilance
is essential throughout pregnancy to ensure the birth of
healthy children.

General Responsibilities

Since this subject is so large I will merely suggest

certain sensible precautions by young and old to avoid
oncological diseases.   I have mentioned the risk of asbestos
exposure, but there are others, including vinyl chloride and
radioactive substances.   Considerable attention is being
focussed on a group of chemicals, which are potent carcinogens
for the urinary system, especially the bladder.   These
compounds are benzidine and naphthylamines, where the
recognition of their risk has led to strict precautions
being taken in their use.

Mankind is exposed to an increasing number of chemicals
in his environment, which are produced in various ways.
For instance, so many chemicals are now used in the
production, preservation and preparation of food.   Constant
testing of these and other chemicals for carcinogenicity is
mandatory to allow appropriate safeguards in their use.
For instance, if a chemical is found to be carcinogenic in
animals, it is wise to eliminate it from human use.   Hormones
are now taken by women on a tremendous scale for various
reasons.   I advise careful observations and monitoring of
any ill-effects during the years ahead, remembering there
may be a latent period of twenty five years before serious
results are seen.   Recently the possibility was considered
that oestrogens may cause endometrial carcinoma; this is
important since many hospitals have established hormone
replacement clinics.

Before closing I make no apology for reiterating the
gravest warning about the tobacco habit responsible for the
present epidemic of tobacco cancers.   Young people are
advised strongly not to start smoking tobacco.   Smokers
have been warned repeatedly of their cancer risk, but,
whilst many doctors have stopped smoking, there seems to be
little public response to this appeal.   If people had the
will, they would surely find the way to give it up,
for even those who were heavily addicted have succeeded.
The cost in poor health and loss of life is so great, I am
convinced we must move to the voluntary abolition of tobacco.
In the meantime the availability of tobacco and the
opportunities to smoke it should regulate its use to a
minimum.   The prevention of these tobacco cancers will be
one of the greatest triumphs of preventive medicine.   This
provides us to-day with a bright hope for the future.

DISCUSSION

Question 1.   Alcohol and Cancer – comments please.

Answer.   Dr. Roe: People who drink so much alcohol
that they develop cirrhosis of the liver certainly increase
their risk of developing that type of cancer, and there is
some association with the drinking of alcohol and larynx
cancer in France, but I think I should say in comfort that
a little alcohol does not probably do many people much harm,
I hope.

Mr. Raven: There is some evidence to associate the
excessive taking of alcohol with carcinoma of the oesophagus.

Question 2.   Would Mr. Raven comment on the value of
screening for breast cancer – this is for the early diagnosis
of breast cancer?

Answer.   The best screening for breast cancer is by
xerography and mammography.   We can diagnose breast cancer
before the tumour can be felt, as small as 0.5 centimetres.
This advance is comparable, I think, in some ways with the
E.M.I. scanner systems.   It is a most valuable method of
early diagnosis of breast cancer .

Question 3.   What suggestions can Mr. Raven make for
sedation in the emaciated patient where vomiting is so often
persistent and injection therapy so very painful in itself.

Answer.   Vomiting is a very important and distressing
symptom in many patients with malignant diseases.   These
patients should be investigated, if possible, to find the
cause of the vomiting.   For example, the electrolyte
imbalances of the body can cause severe vomiting, and the
best treatment is to correct the metabolic disorder.
Prof. Lant, you will recall, stressed the fact that in
hypercalcaemia vomiting is a most important and distressing
symptom, and the way to deal with that cause of vomiting is
to correct the hypercalcaemia by giving oral or intravenous
phosphate or mythromycin intravenously, together with
intravenous fluids.   The point I want to make is that it is
important to find the cause of vomiting whenever possible.
There is a useful range of anti-emetics and anti-nauseants,
which include maxolon, stelazine and stemetil.

Question 4.   We are now in no doubt that cigarette
smoking is a major factor in the cause of lung cancer.
The efforts of governments over the last twenty or so years
leaves much to be desired in this area.   We still find in
our morning papers one page devoted to their advertisements –
with a line at the bottom, "Every packet carries a health
warning!"   Is this not nonsensical?   Can the medical
profession get together with the government to work out
some solution?   Is enough done to discourage young people
from starting this very dangerous habit?

There is also a linked question here.   Why are the
dangers of tobacco not taught in schools where often 90% of
pupils of age 13 – 16 are heavy smokers?

Answer.   There is increasing educational work being
done in schools regarding this particular habit connected
with lung cancer.   The medical profession is working, I
believe, to dissuade people from taking it up.   For example,
the Royal College of Physicians published an admirable
report about the subject some time ago.   As individuals,
we are constantly speaking about it, trying to curtail the
dangerous habit.   There is an association called Ash, which
is very active in this field.   Much work is, therefore,
being done, but I agree with the questioner that more
effective action is required.   I believe we must move
towards the total abolition of tobacco from the world, on a
voluntary basis in the first place.   Let us educate people
to move forward to this accomplishment voluntarily.   If
this is not successful, then I think that other measures
must be taken.   Tobacco should be made nearly impossible
to acquire.   Its price could be raised still further and
the public facilities in which it can be smoked should be
reduced to a bare minimum.

Question 5.   In view of the number of different
treatments now available for cancer, why is the death-rate
rising annually?

Answer.   That is a very important problem to consider.
An important reason in our country, and also elsewhere, is
the tremendous increase in deaths annually from carcinoma of
the lung.   In this disease the results from treatment
remain poor because so many patients are seen with advanced
disease.   Some forms of cancer are falling in incidence,

like stomach cancer in the U.K. and the U.S.A.   Breast
cancer remains a dangerous disease in women.   There are
important advances in treatment but much more work is
required to get patients to come for screening and early
diagnosis.   The best chance for a patient is the treatment
of early disease.   More emphasis on prevention is also
necessary.

Dr. Roe: If I may add a supplement to that, I think
there are two aspects of lung cancer rates.   One is whether
the actual age standardised rates are increasing or falling
and the other, of course, is whether alternative causes of
death, other than cancer, are being prevented more successfully
than those of cancer.   I believe it is true that, apart from
cancer of the lung, there are some real increases, that is
age standardised death-rates, for cancer of the pancreas and
the urinary bladder, but the age standardised death-rate for
cancer of the stomach is falling.   For most other cancers
the age standardised rates are more or less the same.   So,
in other words, although the actual numbers of deaths per
year are increasing, the risk of dying at any particular age
of most cancers, except the ones that are mentioned, lung,
pancreas and bladder, are not increasing.

Question 6.   Are the organisation and facilities
adequate for cancer rehabilitation in the United Kingdom,
since it is now accepted that this work is of the greatest
importance?

Answer.   The Foundation did much pioneer work in this
country in the rehabilitation of the cancer disabled.   This
subject is rightly attracting tremendous interest, not only
in this country but throughout the world.   The philosophy
of the total care of the cancer patient from the time of
diagnosis to resettlement at home and at work has been
accepted and is being translated in a practical way.   I
believe we should give much more attention to this particular
work in our hospitals.   We should have rehabilitation units
in the departments of oncology where all aspects of
rehabilitation are dealt with to restore the whole patient.
We must remember the spiritual requirements of patients as
well as their physical disabilities.   The latter require
skilled physiotherapy, the help of the stomal therapist,
nutritionist, prosthetist and other members of the oncology
team.   The patients with major paralyses caused by cancer
have important problems, - the paraplegics, hemiplegics and

the quadriplegics.   All these patients are suffering
tremendously, and we need special expertise to help them.
I wish to stress the need for several special units in this
country for the treatment of patients with major cancer
paralyses.   All this work of rehabilitation needs to be
greatly expanded and special units and centres are desirable.

Question 7.   Does Mr. Raven see ways in which surgical
treatment can be made more effective than it is to-day?

Answer.   The effectiveness of surgical treatment is
very considerable for many thousands of patients are cured.
The best chance for a patient with a cancerous disease is
early diagnosis and treatment, and this is fundamental where
surgery is concerned.

In some patients better results are obtained with
combination treatment by surgery, radiotherapy and
chemotherapy.   These treatments are combined in different
ways according to the indications.   The greater use of
chemicals with surgery holds out considerable promise for
the future.   Important advances are being made.

Question 8.   Are there important developments in the
surgical treatment of cancer?

Answer.   Technical surgery for cancer has reached a
high standard of perfection.   Anaesthesia, skilled nursing
and the use of post-operative recovery wards and intensive
care units have helped greatly.   In addition, antibiotics
and replacement therapy for blood and electrolytes with the
constant monitoring of patients is very important.

The surgical staging of various oncological diseases,
such as Hodgkin's disease, is an important advance because
the exact treatment can be given for the particular stage.
An important advance is combination treatment where the
surgical operation is part of the whole treatment which
includes radiotherapy and chemotherapy.

Question 9.   Is there anything new available to
counteract the appalling smell of disintegrating cancerous
tissue, as in the last stages of cancer of the breast.
This can be so very distressing and embarrassing for both
patient and family.

Answer.   The usual wound and room deodorants should
be used and frequent dressing of the tumour is also helpful.
Chlorophyll preparations are useful for local application.

Question 10.   Two recent papers in the Lancet prescribed
the use of BCG in treatment of carcinoma of the lung.   Would
a member of the panel kindly explain on this therapy.

Answer.   BCG is being used in the treatment of a number
of tumours, but it must be clearly understood that much more
work on immunology is required before we can really speak
about cancer immunotherapy.   It has been suggested that there
must be only a few tumour cells for BCG to be effective and
the patient's condition is competent to develop an immune
response.   One effect of BCG is to activate macrophage cells
to attack the tumour cells.   Much more information is
required to enable us to understand these mechanisms of
action.

Question 11.   I would like to know why patients with
cancer are so rarely told their diagnosis, when they are told
they have myasthenia gravis, etc., which, as the name implies,
is as serious.   Is it fear that patients will not be able to
cope if they know their diagnosis?

Answer.   Everyone speaks about cancer much more freely
nowadays, which is very helpful.   I believe it is right for
patients to know their diagnosis unless there is some
compelling reason against this.   But they should be told
about their condition kindly and sympathetically in the
presence of a near relative.   At the same time they must be
given hope with the assurance that everything possible will
be done to help them.   Many patients desire to know the
truth about their illness and it is much easier to care for
them when they know and co-operate.   Of course, the word,
cancer, has no scientific meaning and has caused much fear
in the past.   I would substitute the term, oncological
diseases, which are master-minded by the multidisciplinary
subject of oncology.

Question 12.   Has anything been discovered to help the
patient fight his own cancer?

Answer.   The patient's resistance against cancer is
concerned with the immunological reactions connected with

malignant diseases.   There is considerable research
proceeding concerning this important subject, including
finding methods to enhance the patient's reactions in the
hope that malignant cells will be killed.   To bolster up
these reactions the patient's general condition must be kept
as good as possible, including rectifying anaemia and
electrolyte imbalances, treating infections, and maintaining
nutrition, etc.

Question 13.   Is sufficient attention being given to
the possible cancer risks to the developing child in utero?

Answer.   Increasing attention is being given to these
cancer risks in the unborn child.   Since a number of
children are born with cancer and others develop this soon
after birth, the malignant changes took place in utero.
The subjects of uterine carcinogenesis and transplacental
carcinogenesis are of great importance because we know that
the foetus is thereby exposed to a number of environmental
carcinogens.

No pregnant woman should smoke tobacco and she should
take drugs for illness only on the doctor's advice.

CANCER DIAGNOSIS AND THE E.M.I. SCANNER

Richard Hayward

Department of Neurosurgery
Atkinson Morley's Hospital
London

INTRODUCTION

In this review I would like to describe the system of computerised tomography (C.T. scanning) as represented by the EMI scanner. Its original development was for the investigation of all structural abnormalities in the head, but here I will try and place in context the revolutionary effect it has had on the diagnosis and management of intracranial tumours. From this neurological experience, it is possible to predict the effect that computerised tomography will have for other specialities when whole body scanning becomes generally available.

HISTORICAL BACKGROUND
(New, P.F.J. and Scott, W.R. 1975)

The use of X-rays for diagnosis in medicine involves passing a beam of photons through the required target and measuring the resulting geography of X-ray absorption on a suitably sensitised film or screen. Two factors impair the efficiency of this system.

(a) The overall sensitivity must depend on that of the film or screen, and

(b) The rays are passing in a straight line through a target which consists of many structures of differing density.

In this way the eventual effect of each small part of the
X-ray beam will be a reflection of the individual effects of
many superimposed hard and soft tissues.   The process can
be made more sensitive by rotating both the X-ray source and
the film in relation to each other so that the resulting
picture is of a slice of tissue in the target, the information
from above and below having been blurred out by movement.
This process is known as tomography.

Most malignant tumours are soft tissue and can be
visualised by plain X-rays only when their density is in
marked contrast to the surrounding structures, (i.e., a solid
bronchial carcinoma surrounded by air-filled lung).
Radiological diagnosis of cancer often depends on the
introduction of a contrast medium (barium, air, iodine
containing solutions, etc.) which will allow visualisation
of the outside or inside of the relevant organs.

Computerised tomography, as we know it to-day, was
developed at EMI by Mr. Godfrey Hounsfield (Hounsfield, G.N.
1973) and a prototype completed with the co-operation of the
Department of Health and Social Security in August, 1970.
The first machine was installed at Atkinson Morley's Hospital
in 1971 and its clinical development co-ordinated by Dr. James
Ambrose (Ambrose, J.A. 1973).   In the EMI scanner, a thin
beam of photons from a conventional X-ray source moves in a
straight line across the axial plane of the head.   The
photons that emerge are recorded not on film, but by sodium
iodide crystal detectors and the information stored on a
computer.   The whole system of X-ray source and detectors
is linked by a gantry so that they move in parallel.   After
one sweep across the head, this gantry is rotated through
one or more degrees and the process repeated.   The scanning
unit passes through a minimum of 180 degrees and from the
many thousands of readings by the detector, the computer is
able to calculate the amount of photons absorbed by each
individual piece of tissue within the slice of the head that
has been studied.   The resulting information is presented
by the computer as a paper print-out with individual numbers
for the co-efficients of absorption in each block of tissue,
so that mathematically, the head has been treated as a grid
or matrix.   For convenience the same information can be used
to produce an image on a cathode ray tube, where high
densities, such as bone, appear white and low densities, such
as air and water, appear as black.   The resulting image can

easily be photographed on polaroid film so that an immediate
record is available.

The head is ideally suited for development of this system
because the high density of the skull prohibits any direct
radiological visualisation of the soft tissues inside.   It
has become accepted practice to outline the intracranial
structures such as the ventricles and blood vessels, with
contrast media like air, Conray and myodil.   Many of these
techniques are extremely uncomfortable for the patient and
require him to remain still for long periods of time.   For
this reason many of them are carried out under a general
anaesthetic.   Cerebral angiography, encephalography and
ventriculography all have a small, but definite, morbidity
and mortality.   It is not surprising, therefore, that
development of a system which provides as much, or even more,
information as the previous techniques and is free from their
dangers, has been taken up with such enthusiasm.

SCANNING TECHNIQUE

The patient is required to lie on a special couch, the
height and position of which can easily be changed.   The
head is placed, with the neck flexed, within the machine.
In the original EMI scanners, scanning was carried out with
the head (from the supra-orbital to sub-occipital regions)
enclosed within a bag containing water.   With the new
scanners this is no longer necessary and the patient's head
is merely supported by a rest positioned at the cranio-
cervical junction and held steady by a "bean bag".   Scanning
and processing time depend on the type and modifications of
the equipment used, but the latest CT1010 scanner can complete
a "run" in sixty seconds and start to present the information
from two adjacent slices through the head ten seconds later.
The technique is completely non-invasive and can be undertaken
by the patient without risk.   It has now become our custom
in patients suspected of harbouring intracranial tumours to
repeat the scan following the intravenous injection of 60cc
of sodium iothalamate (Conray 420), as it has been clearly
shown from several studies that the quality and quantity of
information about cerebral tumours can be increased greatly
by this technique (Ambrose, J.A., Gooding, M. and Richardson,
A.E., 1975).

PRESENT ROLE OF C.T. SCANNING IN THE DIAGNOSIS
AND MANAGEMENT OF INTRACRANIAL TUMOURS

Soon after the introduction of the EMI scanner it
became obvious that it was going to play a major role in
the diagnosis of a wide spectrum of intracranial disease
(Paxton, R. and Ambrose, J.A. 1974).   Any new diagnostic
technique for use in the field of malignant disease will be
judged by the following criteria:

(1)   Are more tumours being diagnosed since the
      introduction of the technique?

(2)   Is more pre-operative information being
      gathered with regard to (a) pathology, and
      (b) anatomy of the lesions?

(3)   Are other investigations used less?

(4)   Does it represent an improvement in patient
      morbidity and mortality?

(5)   Can tumours be diagnosed at an earlier stage?
      (See Summary)

(1)   Frequency of Cancer Diagnosis

The answer to this question is given in Table 1.   It
can be seen that, although there are fluctuations in both
the numbers of operations for malignant brain tumour and of
patients diagnosed with this condition each year, there does
not appear to be a significant correlation between the
figures before **and after** the introduction of the scanner
into whole-time clinical use (1973).

(2)   (a)   Pathological Information

It is difficult to compare the figures for pre-
operative diagnosis from C.T. scanning and from other
radiological tests because the breadth of information
available from the C.T. scan is so great that no other
single investigation comes close to equalling it.   Air
encephalography and ventriculography provide information
only about the anatomical distortion of the c.s.f. spaces
in the head and do not usually contribute to a pathological

Table 1.   Details of patients investigated and treated for malignant cerebral tumours at Atkinson-Morley's Hospital, 1972 – 1975.

Year	Craniotomies for malignant tumour *	Total No. of malignant tumours diagnosed	No. without histological verification	Total No. of patient admissions
1972	115	284	46	1752
1973	138	214	26	1833
1974	123	248	36	1755
1975	121	296	57	1778

* Glioma and Metastasis.

diagnosis.   A radio-isotope brain scan can only provide
this information, (a) when it shows multiple lesions, which
are probably metastatic, and, (b) when the area of abnormal
uptake is very "hot" and the tumour is likely to be a
meningioma.   Cerebral angiography demonstrates the
distortion of normal intracranial vascular structures, but,
when the tumour has a pathological circulation, it can
supply information about tumour type.   In a recent study
of two hundred supra-tentorial tumours at this hospital,
investigated by arteriography, one hundred and forty-nine
showed evidence of pathological circulation, while forty-one
showed only a mass effect with displacement of the local
vascular pattern (Ambrose, J.A., Gooding, M. and Richardson,
A.E., 1976).   Having identified a pathological circulation,
it is usually possible to differentiate a benign from a
malignant tumour, although well-described areas of confusion
exist between the two.

(2)   (b)   Anatomical Localisation

With regard to tumour position, rectilinear isotope
brain scanning was clearly positive with accurate
localisation in only one hundred and seventy-six cases out
of the two hundred and seventy investigated by this
technique.   In addition, there were forty-eight cases where
a definite false negative result was demonstrated.   Cerebral
angiography revealed ten false negatives out of the two
hundred examined, and the presence of a pathological
circulation in one hundred and forty-nine cases naturally
provided accurate anatomical localisation.   Pneumo-
encephalography has been less commonly performed for tumour
investigation,but was able to provide accurate anatomical
information in seventeen cases out of a total of twenty-one,
these figures being biased because the technique was used
most frequently to localise tumours in the supra-sella
region, an area where its results are extremely good.

C.T. scanning provides useful information concerning
the pathology of cerebral tumours, and in the recent study
it was possible to predict that a tumour was meningioma,
metastases or astrocytoma with accuracies of sixty-seven,
seventy-six and eighty per cent respectively.   When the
scans were reviewed in order to separate infiltrating
lesions (gliomas and metastases) from localised lesions,
the accuracy rose to ninety per cent.   Anatomical

localisation of supratentorial tumours by C.T. scanning
has risen as experience with the technique has increased
and the machinery became more sophisticated.   Using 160 x
160 matrix and tumour enhancement with sodium iothalamate,
the accuracy rate is approaching one hundred per cent
(Ambrose, J.A. et al 1975).

(3) Effect of C.T. Scanning on Other Investigations

Our policy at the present time is to operate on
suspected malignant cerebral tumours after performing only
EMI and radio-isotope scans.   Analysis of fifty consecutive
craniotomies performed until the 16th March, 1976, revealed
that seven patients had a unilateral carotid angiogram
performed before surgery and one patient had a burrhole
biopsy.   Similar analysis of fifty patients operated on at
the same time of the year in 1972 revealed that thirty-two
patients were subjected to angiography and two of them had
more than one major vessel examined.   A further patient
also had a preliminary burrhole biopsy before proceeding to
craniotomy (Hayward, R.D. 1976).   In addition to those
patients eventually shown to have cerebral tumours, there
are many more referred for investigations in whom cerebral
angiography was necessary in order to exclude the presence
of a space-occupying lesion.   In these patients the EMI
scan is more satisfactory as a screening procedure and
cerebral angiography is no longer a routine part of their
investigation.

(4) Patient Mortality and Morbidity

Computerised tomography has carried no significant
mortality or morbidity in this unit.   It has been of
advantage both to the patient and the clinician to
substitute for the many procedures that may require
hospitalisation and general anaesthesia, an investigation
which is non-invasive and which may be performed on an
out-patient basis.   Indeed, these factors carry one
disadvantage as they may tempt clinicians to submit their
patients to neuro-radiological investigations at too low a
threshold of clinical suspicion.   It is not always easy to
divide the available scanning time so that there remains
opportunity, both for the investigation of patients in need

of urgent neurosurgical care and those referred for routine
tumour screening.

FUTURE DEVELOPMENTS

It is not hard to imagine that, as whole body scanning
becomes more available, it will start to fulfil many of the
criteria proposed earlier.   In many parts of the body there
exist already satisfactory and simple methods of cancer
diagnosis, and it will not be necessary to replace them with
computerised tomography.   However, there are other areas
where present day diagnostic methods are often inaccurate,
highly complex and where the patient may still be submitted
to diagnostic surgery.   The evaluation of lesions affecting
the pancreatic gland, for example, may involve endoscopy
with retrograde catheterisation of the pancreatic duct,
complex radio-isotope scanning and selective angiography, in
addition to plain radiographs and barium studies.   Space-
occupying lesions of the kidney revealed by intravenous
pyelography can require arteriography, percutaneous cyst
puncture and even exploration before they are diagnosed as
benign or malignant.   Because C.T. scanning requires
immobility of the tissues examined, it will be particularly
in these retro-peritoneal spaces where it will replace so
many other investigations.

Knowledge of individual tissue densities can be of use
not only for diagnostic purposes, but also for planning and
control of radiotherapy.   The information from the C.T.
scan is precisely what is required to insure that an
effective dose of irradiation at the target site is not
achieved at the expense of the adjacent tissues.

SUMMARY

The introduction of C.T. scanning has brought about a
revolution in the practice of neurology and neurosurgery.
I have emphasised its role in the diagnosis of malignant
tumours of the brain, but it has had a similar impact upon
the management of head injuries, cerebral abscess,
intracranial haemorrhage, hydrocephalus, orbital tumours
and with the newer machines, lesions of the cranio-cervical
junction and upper cervical spine.

Malignant tumours of the central nervous system, whether primary or secondary, usually present with short histories of advancing clinical signs. For this reason, C.T. scanning is unlikely to be responsible for shortening of the time before a definitive diagnosis can be made. Instead, research into finding more effective means of therapy can continue more easily now that diagnosis and localisation have been simplified by a technique that is non-invasive and can also be used in post-operative assessment and follow-up.

REFERENCES

Ambrose, J.A. 1973. Computerised transverse axial scanning - clinical application. British Journal of Radiology 46: 1023-1047.

Ambrose, J.A., Gooding, M.R., Richardson, A.E. 1975. Sodium iothalamate as an aid to diagnosis of intracranial lesions by computerised transverse axial scanning. Lancet ii:669-674.

Ambrose, J.A., Gooding, M.R., Richardson, A.E. 1976. An assessment of the accuracy of computerised transverse axial scanning (EMI scanner) in the diagnosis of intracranial tumour - a review of 366 patients. Brain 98:569-582.

Hayward, R.D. 1976. Personal observation.

Hounsfield, G.N. 1973. Computerised transverse axial scanning - description of system. British Journal of Radiology 46:1016-1022.

New, P.F.J., Scott, W.R. 1975. Computerised tomography of the brain and orbit (EMI scanning). Williams and Wilkins Company, Baltimore, Maryland.

Paxton, R., Ambrose, J.A. 1974. A brief review of the first 650 patients. British Journal of Radiology 47:530-565.

DISCUSSION

Question 1.   Since the E.M.I. scanner is of immense value in the diagnosis of brain tumours, is this facility available in the major centres in the United Kingdom?

Answer.   There is an increasing number of scanners going in all over the country at present.   In the London region

there are five, two at the Atkinson Morley's Hospital in
Wimbledon, two at the National Hospital, Queen Square, and
another at the Wellington Hospital.   Most of the major
neurological centres in England and Wales are now getting
the E.M.I. scanners.   These are all head scanners.   There
are three whole body (general purpose) scanners working now.

Question 2.   (a) How great is the exposure of the
patient to radiation in the E.M.I. scanner, and, (b) is the
method used serially?

Answer.   It looked from the illustrations I was showing
that there would be a great deal of irradiation involved in
each scan.   In fact, each individual beam of X-rays is very
small and the total exposure is slight.   To do an EMI scan
on the present equipment involves three or four 'cuts' of the
head and uses less irradiation than a conventional series of
skull X-rays.   The irradiation dose, however, is increasing
as the resolution of the scanner becomes greater and at
present, per cut, per slice, of the head the irradiation on
the new E.M.I. CT 1010 is probably two rads.

With regard to serial scanning: yes, we do use it
serially, particularly when treating patients with cerebral
tumours without actually operating.   As many of you know,
symptoms caused by brain metastases can often be alleviated
by giving the patients high doses of steroids, such as
Dexamethasone.   We tend to follow up these patients using
the CT scan to see if we can monitor any difference in the
configuration of the tumour and the surrounding oedema of
the brain after they have been improved by steroids.

Question 3.   Does Mr. Hayward consider that the E.M.I.
scanner will prove of equal importance in other organs of
the body?

Answer.   Yes, I am sure it will.   The disadvantages
of scanning the rest of the body, as opposed to the head, is
that the scanning systems cannot deal with movements of the
patient.   If you are taking a conventional X-ray, it is
over in a fraction of a second and, as you know, the picture
can be blurred by movement.   These CT scans go on for
several seconds - maybe even a minute or more, and they can
be completely ruined by movement.   In the head that is no
problem if the patient will keep still.   In the rest of the

body though you have a variety of other physiological
movements which distort the scans.   For instance, it is
impossible to look at the inside of the heart with the
present scanners because of the heart beats.   That may be
possible in the future but it is not now.   Breathing can be
overcome by asking the patient to hold the breath and most
can do so with a little practice for twenty seconds, which is
the current scan time of the E.M.I. general purpose scan.
In the abdomen there is continual peristaltic activity, which
can impair the quality of the scans.   The patients are
usually given something to stop gut motility prior to the
scan.   From what I have been saying, I think it is most
likely that the organs which will be shown best on the whole
body scanner, and therefore make the biggest contribution,
are the organs which have no natural movement of their own.
I am thinking particularly of the mediastinum which is
extremely difficult to look at, at the present time, and also
of the retroperitoneal tissues.

At the same time the manufacturers are working hard to
reduce the time involved with each scan and some of the newer
prototypes can complete a cut in five seconds.

When the distorting movement is regular in frequency,
as with the heart, it may be possible to build up a complete
scan from individual readings that have been taken at only
one phase of the cardiac cycle.   This would then produce an
apparently stationary picture.   This system would be
analogous to taking a cine film of a rotating wheel.   If
the speed of rotation and the speed of the film are exactly
synchronised, then the eventual image will be of a wheel
that appears stationary.

HEALTH, NUTRITION AND METABOLISM IN MALIGNANT DISEASE

Ariel F. Lant

Professor of Clinical Pharmacology and
Therapeutics
Westminster Hospital Medical School, London

Current clinical management of the patient with cancer
involves a multidisciplinary approach which utilizes the
resources of surgery, radiotherapy, chemotherapy,
immunotherapy, and includes last but not least, supportive
management.   It is often not realised how much demand is
made upon the individual by the various intensive treatments
we employ to treat neoplastic disease.   Supportive therapy
encompasses a number of in-patient aspects of management,
which may not only have the capacity to improve the general
well-being of the patient but can also boost host resilience
so as to enable standard, though demanding, forms of
treatment to be undertaken.   Where one is dealing with
palliation of advanced terminal cancer, supportive therapy
takes paramount place in alleviating suffering and allowing
the patient to lead as comfortable an existence as possible.

The spectrum of supportive therapy is large and
includes a large number of facets of the malignant disease
process, ranging from relief of pain to the serious hazards
of opportunistic infection or haematological dyscrasias.
In this paper I shall be concentrating primarily on the
nutritional and metabolic problems which can often be
anticipated or reversed by an understanding of the
mechanisms involved.

NEOPLASIA AND NUTRITIONAL DERANGEMENT

Whereas much research has been devoted to the study of

possible associations between environmental factors,
including ingested foodstuffs, and development of tumours,
remarkably little attention has been paid to the profound
influences which tumour growth and extension undoubtedly
exert upon the normal nutritional and metabolic processes of
the body.

It has been recognised for many years that cancer,
irrespective of its site or pathological type, is characterised
by generalised metabolic features of which probably the most
striking is cachexia.   This may be gross, even with the most
localised of tumours.   Initially, weight loss may occur with
adequate or even increased food intake, indicating the
existence of a hypercatabolic state.   This means that the
rate of tissue breakdown greatly exceeds that of tissue
synthesis.   As the tumour progresses, anorexia develops and
there is associated malabsorption of foodstuffs from the
gastro-intestinal tract.   The net effect of these developments
is massive wasting of body tissues.

Several factors contribute to this sequence of events and
can be related to changes in metabolism of the three major
groups of nutrient.

PROTEIN

A malignant tumour which is growing rapidly may
preferentially "trap" protein within it at a time when other
body tissues are wasting.   Protein intake which is adequate
for nitrogen balance in normal people becomes inadequate for
the cancer patient.   In other words, the normal tissues of
the body provide the building blocks for synthesis of more
tumour.   Provision of an abundant supply of readily
assimilable nitrogen and calories can help to replete host
tissues.   Often, however, the process of repletion is
incomplete because substances may be produced by the tumour
which prevent the attainment of a balanced state.   Such
substances may exert effects on remote tissues by inhibiting
tissue synthesis and also encouraging greater loss of
nitrogen in urine and faeces.

CARBOHYDRATE

The most readily appreciated evidence of disturbed

carbohydrate metabolism in man is the level of blood glucose and its spillover into urine.   Normally, circulating glucose levels are regulated within close limits around 70-100 mg./100 ml. (4-6 mmol/litre) due to the maintenance of a dynamic equilibrium between processes aimed at raising or lowering the blood level.   These are depicted in Table 1.   Decreased glucose tolerance is common in patients with cancer and fasting as well as post-prandial blood glucose levels may be abnormally high.   The reasons are not fully understood though it is likely that diminished tissue responsiveness to endogenous insulin may play a part. Where adrenal cortico-steroids are being administered in therapy, or being produced in abnormal amounts endogenously, these may be a cause, but often no obvious hormonal abnormality can be detected.

Table 1.   Regulation of Blood Glucose.

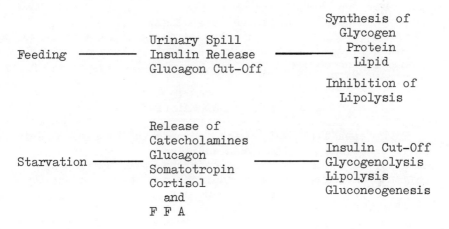

LIPID

It is common to find at operation, or at autopsy, in cancer patients, a gross depletion of body fat, such as for example, in subcutaneous or retroperitoneal tissues.   Again, although the mechanisms are not fully worked out, experimental evidence from animal tumour systems suggests that certain tumours produce lipid-mobilising substances which cause diffuse breakdown of stored fat (lipolysis) from tissue depots.

CACHEXIA

Cachexia of cancer is a broad-based entity which ranges
on the one hand from the patient with an undiagnosed neoplasm,
who consults his doctor on account of a minor degree of
weight loss, to the patient with terminal disease, who has
gross muscle wasting and weakness.

Cancer cells have a remarkable capacity for capturing
from the internal environment and concentrating all the
nutrients necessary for their continued growth at the expense
of other body tissues.   The way in which this is achieved
is still unclear.   Tumours produce a variety of enzymes
which circulate and can exert their effects on local or
remote tissues.   Thus, for example, local release of the
enzyme, hyaluronidase, may assist in malignant invasiveness.
Increased production of lysosomal enzymes may contribute to
the phenomenon of cachexia.   Further, by-products of tumour
metabolism which have potent hormonal properties, may exert
widespread effects on tissue metabolism.   Such ectopic
hormones or enzymes may be synthesized by neoplastic tissue
or, in some cases, may merely represent leakage of metabolites
from dying cancer cells.

CANCER THERAPY AND MALNUTRITION

The catabolic state which features in the cancer patient,
may undergo exaggeration when additional burdens of major
surgery, radiotherapy, or chemotherapy, are superimposed.
Patients who have recently undergone any form of elective
surgical procedure, are starving, not only because of the
necessary pre-operative withdrawal of oral nutrition, but
also because they display an accelerated catabolic response
to the operation.   Even if the malignancy is anatomically
resectable, negative nitrogen balance, lowered host resistance,
with impaired capacity for wound healing, may militate
against either operability or fitness to withstand any other
form of anti-tumour treatment.

Similarly, the patient who is receiving cytotoxic
chemotherapy and/or a course of radiotherapy, may have severe
metabolic illness, added to which apprehension and mental
depression may further inhibit those hypothalamic areas of
mid-brain which control appetite.   Stimulation of the

chemoreceptor trigger zone and vomiting centre in the medulla
serves to generate the nausea, vomiting, and aversion to
food, which so often characterises this group of patients.

NUTRITIONAL DEFICIENCY AND DRUG THERAPY

Malnutrition can arise during chronic therapy with a
number of drugs commonly used either as part of a composite
cytotoxic chemotherapy regime, or as adjuvant treatment aimed
at control of coincidental disorders, such as, for example,
cardiac or hepatic failure.

Raised levels of circulating corticosteroids may be
produced, either through stimulation of the patient's own
adrenals, or through intentional use of powerful synthetic
glucocorticoids, such as, prednisolone or dexamethasone, in
treatment.   Prolonged tissue exposure to such substances
leads to general protein breakdown with osteoporosis and the
risk of attendant bony fracture.   Urinary losses of potassium,
the major cation within cells, occurs and this produces a
clinical state of lethargy and muscle weakness.   Urinary
potassium wastage is also a common sequel of therapy with
oral diuretics, such as, "loop" compounds or benzothiadiazines
(thiazides).   Where dietary intake of potassium-containing
foods is inadequate, this constitutes a significant hazard,
especially if digitalis glycosides are also being administered,
as their effects are exaggerated.   Less common effects of
benzothiadiazines include hypercalcaemia and hypomagnesaemia
(see below).

Many of the cytotoxic drugs employed in cancer
chemotherapy are gastro-intestinal irritants, leading to
nausea, vomiting and diarrhoea.   This may be due to local
effects on the gastro-intestinal mucosa, or through central
effects exerted via the medulla and vagus nerve.   Where such
drug therapy has to be continued, the ensuing reduction in
food intake and loss of valuable minerals and fluid may be of
considerable importance in undermining any beneficial effect
of the treatment on the cancer process.   Patients often
stop their therapy to avoid unwanted effects;   yet often,
such drug induced toxicity can be minimised by carefully
planning dosage to suit individual patients' needs.   The
regimen can be tailored to maintain a level of therapeutic
effectiveness and, at the same time, remain acceptable to

the patient.   Much more knowledge is needed of the
pharmacokinetics of cytotoxic drugs so as to allow the
attending doctor to predict likely exaggeration of drug
effects, potential interaction with other drugs in the
presence of disease in key organs involved in the normal
processes of detoxification, such as, for example, the liver
or kidneys.

In certain instances, disturbed metabolism may be an
inseparable component of the cellular mode of action of the
particular therapeutic attack.   Thus methotrexate causes
folic acid deficiency and, through this, reduction in cellular
DNA and RNA - effects which interfere with growth of such
tumours as choriocarcinoma and certain types of leukaemia.
Hyperuricaemia and secondary gout may result from release of
cellular purines in myeloproliferative disorders or lymphomas
being treated with antileukaemia drugs or radiotherapy.

DERANGEMENT IN MINERAL METABOLISM

Probably the commonest derangement of mineral metabolism
associated with cancer is hypercalcaemia which can occur with
or without the presence of bone metastases.   The clinical
picture is non-specific and may involve many systems. (Fig. 2)
In severe cases, the condition may present with intractable
vomiting, profound weakness, severe dehydration and acute
deterioration in renal function, progressing rapidly to coma
and death.   The hypercalcaemia is largely due to imbalance
between the normal processes of bone resorption and deposition
and is most readily explicable when there is widespread
destruction of bone, such as, in secondary involvement by
carcinoma or multiple myeloma.   However, some cases of
hypercalcaemia occur without any evidence of bone metastases.
The condition is then referred to as ectopic hyperparathyroidism
Here the abnormality is usually due to synthesis and secretion
of a parathormone (PTH)-like substance by the malignant tumour,
commonly of the lung or kidney.

Whatever the cause, the hypercalcaemic state requires
urgent management.   Rehydration with substantial volumes of
intravenous saline may suffice as an initial measure but, on
a chronic basis, the most useful treatment is the use of
inorganic phosphate, which is available commercially in a
number of oral preparations and as a liquid for intravenous

Table 2.   Clinical Features of Hypercalcaemia.

Gastro-intestinal	Anorexia
	Nausea and vomiting
	Peptic ulcer
	Acute pancreatitis
Urinary	Polyuria and polydipsia
	Renal insufficiency
	Nephrocalcinosis
Neurological	Fatigue and muscle weakness
	Depression; psychotic behaviour
	Disorientation and coma
Metastatic Calcification	Blood vessels
	Joints
	Eye

use in emergency.   Gastro-intestinal irritation is common
with oral phosphate and so in chronic use the treatment
should be in the lowest effective dose.   If it fails, then
recourse may be had to the cytotoxic substance, mithramycin,
given intravenously.

Chronic diarrhoeal loss of essential minerals must not
be overlooked, as it is not an uncommon accompaniment of
either the malignant process, or the treatment thereof with
drugs or radiotherapy.   As well as potassium depletion,
deficiency of magnesium may occur and be overlooked,
especially as the clinical features of both deficiency states
are similar and vague - apathy and muscular weakness.   By
contrast, it is of interest that active attempts to induce
potassium and magnesium deficiency by dietary means, coupled
with haemodialysis, have been associated with repression of
certain malignant tumours.   This illustrates, yet again,
the complex interplay which exists between the nutritive
requirements for cancer growth and the nutritional
deficiencies and clinical sequelae which can be secondarily

evoked by such growth.

VITAMINS

The major vitamin which has excited much attention in its possible association with neoplastic disease has been ascorbic acid, or vitamin C. Whilst frank clinical scurvy is rare in the United Kingdom, even among the undernourished geriatric population, some of the elderly and patients with chronic debilitating diseases, such as, rheumatoid arthritis, share with cancer patients a significant degree of vitamin C depletion which is frequently subclinical. Evidence has also been adduced for a role of high-dose vitamin C in enhancing tissue resistance to spread of infiltrating malignant tumours. This could reflect another facet of the protective role of the vitamin in altering the balance of the tumour/host relationship in favour of the host.

Another area of interest in the therapeutic potential of ascorbic acid is in treatment of metastatic disease of bone where experimental work has shown in breast carcinoma that raised urinary excretion of the non-essential amino-acid, hydroxyproline, is associated with low levels of leucocyte ascorbic acid. Collagen is the only mammalian protein that contains a significant amount of hydroxyproline and so increased excretion can be used as a marker of bone metabolism. It has been found that increased urinary hydroxyproline in patients with breast carcinoma which has netastasised to bone, can be reversed by administration of high-dose ascorbic acid. The implication of such findings is that the vitamin may slow down the metabolic degradation of collagen associated with proliferation of metastases

DIETARY THERAPY

In the light of this discussion, the importance of adequate nutrition in the patient with malignant disease cannot be overstressed. There is no evidence that a good diet can cure cancer but there is no doubt that it may add considerably to the comfort of the patient. Once the diagnosis has been made and a programme of ablative surgery, irradiation, or cytotoxic drug therapy, has been drawn up, attention should be directed to planning a suitable

supportive diet.   This should have a calorie and nutrient
content which is higher than normal but in a form which is
acceptable to the patient.   The Marie Curie Memorial
Foundation has produced a most useful educational leaflet,
No. 15, entitled, "Diet and Nutrition."   This give practical
guidance on nutritional matters for cancer patients and their
relatives.   Inadequate food intake is not necessarily an
indication for parenteral feeding.   Often patients with
weakness, pain, depression or dysphagia, cannot eat enough
and so they are best helped by a frequent and generous supply
of foods which are appetising and easily swallowed.   If
there is partial or complete obstruction to the functions of
eating, swallowing, or digestion, liquidized feeding may be
required by nasogastric tube, gastrostomy or enterostomy.
Where it is impossible for the patient to receive adequate
nutrition via the gastro-intestinal tract, then parenteral
alimentation becomes essential.

NASOGASTRIC FEEDING

This method can provide all types of natural nutrients
in adequate quantities.   Large amounts of fluid can be given
with relative safety, which is very important where dehydration
is present.   Supplementary materials and drugs, which may be
impalatable, can be given down the tube and there is the added
advantage that feeds can be prepared readily, stored and
administered with ease.   The hazards of tube feeding are, in
general, less than with intravenous feeding, though diarrhoea
may be induced by unsuitably-balanced constituents, such as,
excessively high content of fat, sugar or electrolytes.   At
the same time, it is always important to provide enough water
to allow the kidneys to excrete the ultimate load of solutes
delivered to them, especially end-products of protein and
purine metabolism, such as, urea and uric acid.   Medium
chain triglycerides (MCT) are useful in tube feeding, where
steatorrhoea has been provoked by inclusion of conventional
fats.   Many balanced recipes are available; mostly these
are milk-based, using Complan (Glaxo) or Instant Breakfast
(Carnation) with added glucose,iron and other mineral salts,
vitamins, and methylcellulose as a hydrophilic bulk agent.
Experience has also been expanding in recent years with use
of chemically defined or "elemental" diets, in which there
is very little fat present and the protein source is in the
form of amino-acids with addition of other easily digestible
materials, including minerals and vitamins.

GASTROSTOMY AND ENTEROSTOMY FEEDING

Here, feeding takes place through a tube inserted at operation into the stomach or jejunum. The procedure is simple and can be undertaken with relative simplicity in seriously ill patients. Similar mixtures to those used in nasogastric feeding are employed and the technique may be an invaluable temporary measure aimed at replenishing lost body tissue where malignant disease has made it impossible to pass a nasogastric tube. We have used this approach extensively in preparing patients with, for example, advanced oesophageal carcinoma, for subsequent treatment with intensive irradiation. One word of caution, and this relates to over-enthusiastic carbohydrate administration in tube feeds. Apart from osmotic effects of unabsorbed disaccharides leading to intestinal hurry, rapid entry of high concentrations of glucose into the circulation may induce acute insulin deficiency. There is a risk of inducing a hyperosmolar state with hyperglycaemia but no ketosis, especially in ill patients whose pancreatic insulin reserve may already be inadequate.

INTRAVENOUS FEEDING

Intravenous administration of nutrients bypasses the processes of gastro-intestinal digestion and absorption. It requires the administered foodstuffs to be given, therefore, in a readily assimilable form. Blood and blood products are probably the substances given most frequently by this route to replace either formed elements lost by haemorrhage, or inadequately produced by diseased bone marrow.

Where oral or tube feeding is impossible, intravenous nutrition can be a life-saving measure, as after major operations for malignant diseases of the head and neck, oesophagus or bowel. Usually, it is required to help the patient in a crisis which may last a few days only, but recent experience has shown that it can be used to provide complete nutrition for weeks and even months. Such a situation could arise, for instance, where the gastro-intestinal tract is out of action for a prolonged period after a major resection procedure.

Once decided upon, intravenous nutrition usually
requires the calories to be provided in concentrated form,
either as hypertonic sugar solutions or fat emulsions.
The technical problems of removing pyrogens and preparing
stable emulsions of lipid have been overcome and a number
of safe, though expensive, preparations suitable for
intravenous use are available.   These are derived from
cottonseed oil or soya bean oil.   Nitrogen source solutions
are available as either protein hydrolysates, or mixtures of
synthetic L-amino acids.   Where intravenous lipids are being
given concurrently with amino acid preparations, a "double
drip" technique using a 'Y' tube is conveniently employed.
Glucose is undoubtedly the carbohydrate source of choice,
though concentrated solutions undoubtedly are irritant.
Other carbohydrate energy sources, which are often used,
include the non-insulin dependent sorbitol, or fructose and
ethyl alcohol.   The risk of thrombophlebitis can be
lessened by infusing hypertonic solutions into a central
vein.   Scrupulous aseptic technique is required to avoid
the complication of septicaemia.   However, one of the main
hazards of intravenous feeding is overload of the circulation
so that, whenever employed, no matter for how short a period,
careful monitoring of water and electrolyte balance is
essential.   Carefully handled, the technique can provide the
essential metabolic support needed to allow the patient with
malignant disease to withstand the demands which major
surgery and anti-tumour therapy might make together as part
of a combined effort to eradicate certain types of cancer.

SUMMARY

To speak of health in the context of a patient with
malignant disease may appear a contradiction in terms.
However, the well-being of such patients is the major aim
of all those concerned in managing the cancer problem.
The modern emphasis on an integrated therapeutic approach
has done much to bring together the resources of the various
professions involved in cancer care, so as to provide a
comprehensive programme of treatment which has brought us a
little nearer the solution.

Certain important areas remain where much intensive
research is still needed.   I have endeavoured to emphasise
some of the nutritional and metabolic aspects of cancer,

which still raise questions that cannot be answered, but
deserve serious attention since their solution could
contribute significantly to the conquest of this major
human scourge.

NEWER CHEMICALS FOR CANCER TREATMENT

Iain W.F. Hanham

Consultant in Radiotherapy and Oncology

Westminster Hospital, London

The success of cancer chemotherapy to date has been based largely on empirical observations and results, when any compound has been used successfully to kill selectively tumour cells in a clinical situation.

In an attempt to rationalize the development of cytotoxic agents, the American National Cancer Institute has evaluated a large number of compounds for possible antitumour activity; this figure is now running at 30,000 a year, when synthetic chemical and natural products derived from fermentation processes, or plant and animal sources are tested with a current yield in the ratio 1:40,000 drugs tested, so contributing to the 30 drugs in clinical use.

To-day new drugs undergo a rigorous programme of testing. (Table 1) Eventually a very few drugs are selected for clinical study. Animal models are the initial test tumours, (Table 2) but, although drugs can show a high selectivity in such a system, this is often not readily projected clinically. At the present time the new drugs under study in an attempt to find those most suitable for clinical use are shown in Tables 3, 4, 5 and 6.

Table 1.   Programme for testing new drugs.

In vivo pharmacologic testing

A.   Drug toxicity in normal mice

B.   Drug toxicity in mice with tumours

C.   Pharmacologic determination of effective
     drug levels, for comparison with direct
     measurement of drug levels

Drug activity in a spectrum of tumour systems
In vivo antitumour testing of drugs

A.   Drug effect on tumour growth

B.   Drug effect on survival time of tumourous
     host; schedule and route of administration

C.   Relation of dose-response curves in treated
     tumour-bearing mice to dose-response curves
     in normal mice

D.   Drug effect on tumour cell kill and on cure
     of animals

E.   Intracranial tumour and tumour at other
     sequestered sites

F.   Resistance

G.   Metastasis

H.   Drug action on immune response of host

     1.   Effect of drugs on cell-mediated immunity
     2.   Effect of drugs on host-versus-graft
          reactions
     3.   Effect of drugs on graft-versus-host
          (GVH) reactions
     4.   Effect of drugs on lymphocyte proliferative
          response in vitro
     5.   Effect of drugs on humoral immune responses

I.   Combination chemotherapy

J.   Combined modalities

     1.   Surgery plus chemotherapy
     2.   Immunity plus chemotherapy
     3.   Radiation plus chemotherapy

K.   Special test models

L.   Carcinogenic activity

M.   Chronobiologic influences on drug activity

In vitro characterization of drugs

Application of methodology to selection of analogs

Conclusion

Table 2.   <u>Animal Models</u>.

Leukaemia L1210

Leukaemia P388

Melanoma B16

Lewis Lung Tumour

Ehrlich Ascites

Yoshida Sarcoma

Table 3.   <u>Alkylating Agents</u>.

Iphosphamide

Yoshi-864

Galactitol

Asaley

Table 4.   <u>Antimetabolites</u>

Ftorafur

Baker's Antifol

Cyclocytidine

AAFC (2-2' Anhydro-1-B-D-Arabinofuranosyl-
            5-Fluorocytosine)

Diglycoaldehyde

Table 5.   Antitumour Antibiotics

    Chromomycin A3
    Piperazinedione

    Mitotic Inhibitors

    VM–26
    VP–16

Table 6.   Miscellaneous

    5–Azacytidine
    ICRF 159
    Cis–Platinum (II) Diamminedichloride
    Cytembena

    Two of the most recent important durgs are Adriamycin from Western Europe, and Bleomycin from Japan. (Table 7)

Table 7.   Bleomycin
            Adriamycin

    A spectrum of recent effective chemical agents is shown in Table 8 and Figure 1.

Table 8.   Nitrosoureas

                    BCNU
                    CCNU
                    Methyl CCNU

            Adriamycin
            Bleomycin
            DTIC
            Streptozotocin
            L–Asparaginase

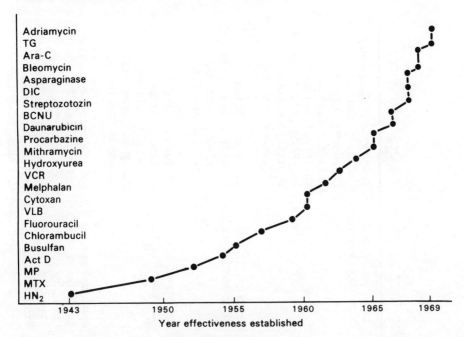

Fig. 1

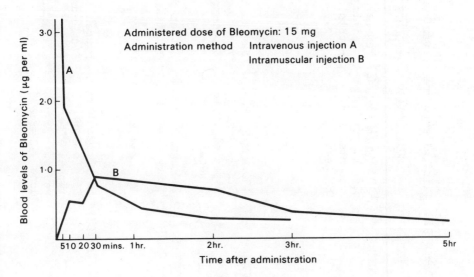

Fig. 2

Table 9.   Clinical spectrum of various chemicals.

DRUG	USUAL DOSAGE	ACUTE TOXICITY	DELAYED	MAJOR INDICATIONS
BCNU	100 mgm/M^2/day x 2 i.v. <u>not</u> to be repeated for 6 weeks	Nausea and vomiting Hepatotoxicity	Leucopenia and thrombocytopenia	Primary and Secondary CNS Neoplasm Hodgkin's Disease Multiple Myeloma Malignant Melanoma Non-Hodgkin's Lymphoma Burkitt's Tumour GI Adenocarcinoma
CCNU	130 mgm/M^2 P.O. Single dose repeated after 6 weeks	Nausea and vomiting Hepatotoxicity	Leucopenia and thrombocytopenia	Hodgkin's Disease Primary & Secondary CNS GI Adenocarcinoma. Bronchial and Renal
METHYL CCNU	200 mgm/M^2 P.O. every 6 weeks	Nausea and vomiting	Leucopenia and thrombocytopenia	GI Adenocarcinoma. Malignant Gliomas Malignant Melanoma Malignant Lymphomas Squamous Carcinoma.
ADRIAMYCIN	$60-90 \text{ mgm/M}^2$ i.v. Single dose repeat after 3 weeks. Total dose 550 mgm/M^2	Nausea Red Urine (**not** haematuria.)	Bone marrow depression Cardiotoxicity Alopecia Stomatitis	Soft Tissue Sarcoma Osteosarcoma Hodgkin's Disease Non-Hodgkin's Disease Breast Carcinoma Bronchial Carcinoma.

Drug	Dose	Toxicity		Indications
BLEOMYCIN	$10-15$ mgm/M^2/wk or twice weekly. i.m. Total dose 180 mgm	Nausea, vomiting fever	Skin reaction Pulmonary fibrosis Stomatitis alopecia Not bone marrow	Hodgkin's Disease Non-Hodgkin's Lymphoma Testicular Radiation Potentiator Squamous Carcinoma Head and Neck. Penis
DTIC (Dacarbazine)	$150-200$ mgm/M^2 daily for 5 days	Nausea and vomiting	Rare bone marrow depression	Malignant Melanoma Hodgkin's Disease Non-Hodgkin's Disease Sarcoma
STREPTOZOTOCIN	$1g/M^2$ weekly i.v. for 4 weeks	Nausea and vomiting	Renal damage	Malignant Insulinoma Carcinoid
L-ASPARAGINASE	10,000 I.U./M^2 alternate day x 4 or weekly	Nausea, fever anaphylaxis	Hepatotoxicity Pancreatitis CNS depression	Acute Lymphatic Leukaemia Non-Hodgkin's Lymphoma

Table 9 shows the agents, dose and clinical spectrum.

Bleomycin is given intramuscularly and remains in
fairly high concentration and is said to have less side
effects when administered in this fashion. (Fig. 2)   It is
a glycopeptide antibiotic and was first used clinically in
1965.   It has particular value in the management of tumours
arising from squamous epithelium.   It was also found to
inhibit DNA repair following radiation damage, and
experimental work with animal models, bacterial, mammalian
cell lines, and DNA itself, have shown an additive
tumouricidal effect, which can be reproduced clinically.

It is non-toxic to the bone marrow, and has been
effectively used in combination treatment of Hodgkin's
disease, non-Hodgkin's lymphoma, and testicular tumours.
It is also useful where marrow infiltration inhibits other
chemotherapy modalities, such as, in bronchial carcinoma.

It is an important compound when used in combination
regimes, particularly in the treatment of Hodgkin's disease,
(Fig. 3) increasing the complete remission rate to 92%, and
in a dose well below the toxic levels.   The original MOPP
regime was the first successful combination of drugs, a
principle which will be referred to later. (Table 10)

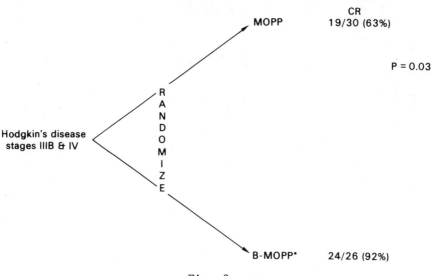

Fig. 3

Table 10.   Remission induction in Hodgkin's disease.   All
             patients had Stage III or IV disease and 76%
             had Stage IVB disease.

Single Agents	No. of Cases	Complete Remission (%)
Prednisone		10
Nitrogen Mustard		10
Cyclophosphamide	389	11
Vincristine	23	13
Vinblastine	88	20
Procarbazine	48	18
Combination Chemotherapy		
COP ●	107	36
MOPP ■		
National Cancer Institute	43	81
Southwest Group	110	72

● Cyclophosphamide, vincristine, prednisone

■ HN_2, vincristine, procarbazine, prednisone

    <u>Adriamycin</u> is an anthracycline antibiotic with the
chemical formula as illustrated. (Fig. 4)

    In contrast to many agents its effectiveness is limited
not only to leukaemia models, but extends to experimental
carcinomas and sarcomas.   It also has a broad clinical
spectrum, as illustrated in Tables 11 and 12.

    The drug has a relatively slow excretion rate, which is
affected by poor liver function.   It also appears to have
relatively specific selective action against tumour cells
compared to normal tissues, and is active against non-cycling
cells (G_0) and, therefore, clinically active against those

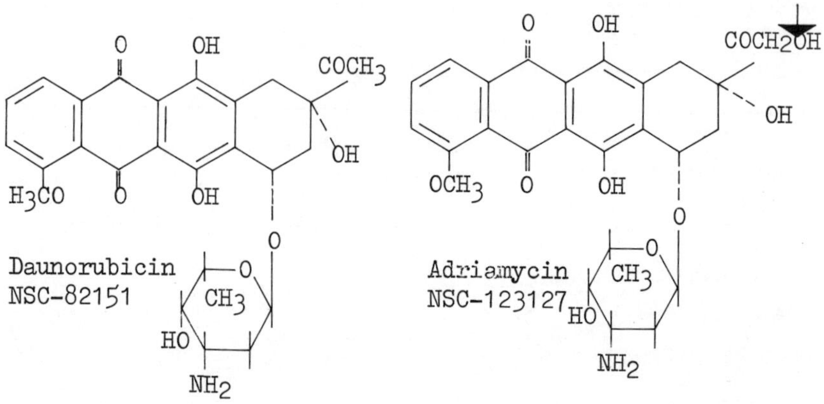

Fig. 4.   Daunorubicin and adriamycin.

Table 11.   Tumours in which adriamycin has demonstrated
definite activity.

Tumour	No. of Cases	Response ■ %
Breast Carcinoma ●	193	37
Sarcoma ●	351	27
Lung Carcinoma	314	22
Oatcell	34	29
Squamous ●	61	36
Adenocarcinoma ●	43	23
Hodgkin's Disease	67	33
Non-Hodgkin Lymphoma ●	94	40
Acute Leukaemia:		
Lymphoblastic	148	24 ▲
Monocytic	57	26 ▲

●Diseases in which adriamycin is definitely or probably
the most active single chemotherapeutic agent.
■Response = 50% decrease in tumour mass.
▲Complete remission.

Table 12.   Tumours in which adriamycin has probable
            activity.

Tumour	No. of Cases	Response %
Testis (non-seminomas)	60	20
Bladder ●	97	28
Cervix ●	28	32
Ovary ●	48	38
Head and Neck squamous	67	19
Thyroid ●	22	45

● Adriamycin is definitely or probably the most active
  single chemotherapeutic agent.

tumours with a low rate of cell turnover.   However, it is
toxic against bone marrow and the hair follicles, which are
normal cells with a high turnover.   The importance of this
drug lies in its broad spectrum of activity, and the potential
of pharmacological modifications of its structure could lead
to greater activity in clinical situations as was seen in the
chemical transformation from Daunorubicin to Adriamycin.

Two compounds which are currently of interest, but not
so established as Bleomycin and Adriamycin are the following:

I.C.R.F. 159

1,2-Di(3,5-dioxopirazine-1-yl) propane

Cis-Platinum (II) Diamminedichloride

Cis-Platinum interferes with DNA synthesis and is one
of a group of platinum compounds exhibiting antitumour
activity in animals.   It is of no value used orally, but
systemically appears effective in lymphomas, and combination
therapy in testicular cancer.

ICRF-159 is a compound which has a selective effect in
animal models, and is administered orally.   Interest was
aroused because it had the curious effect in the Lewis lung
system of preventing metastases by developing normal blood
vessels around the margins of the implant.

It can cause a dramatic reduction in blast cells in the
peripheral blood in leukaemias, but often gives rise to marked
haematological depression.   Clinical useful effects have
been shown in small groups of patients with large bowel cancer,
and squamous carcinoma of the lung.

There is also evidence in animal model systems of the
drug potentiating radiation in comparison with more generally
accepted clinical agents.

The future of any new agent must be considered in the
context of the modern use of drugs, either in combination
regimes, or as adjuvant therapy following primary treatment.
The criteria of using drugs in combination are shown in
Table 13.

Table 13.   SINGLE AGENT ACTIVE AGAINST DISEASE

                     INDEPENDENT ACTION BIOCHEMICALLY

                     DIFFERING CELL CYCLE SPECIFICITIES

                     NO OVERLAP OF TOXICITY

Some of the current 'prophylactic' regimes are
illustrated in Table 14.

However, tumours with a high rate of cell division and
a high rate of cell loss still remain the most sensitive.
Many attempts have been made to control the entry of cells
into mitosis. (Fig. 5)

This shows the cell cycle, and ideally a non-toxic drug
would synchronise the entry of target cells into the
susceptible mitotic phase.   Many drugs can act at different
phases of the cell cycle, but 70% can be in a resting or
non-responsive phase.

Table 14.   'PROPHYLACTIC CHEMOTHERAPY'

    BREAST

L—PAM	Melphalan
C.M.F.	Cyclophosphamide
	Methotrexate
	5 Flouro-uracil

   OSTEOSARCOMA

Vincristine
Methotrexate
Adriamycin

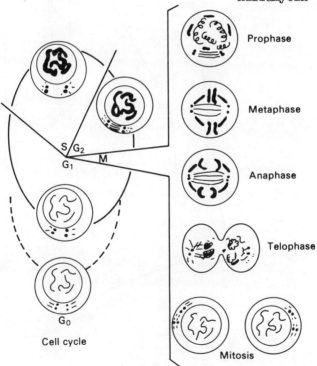

Fig. 5

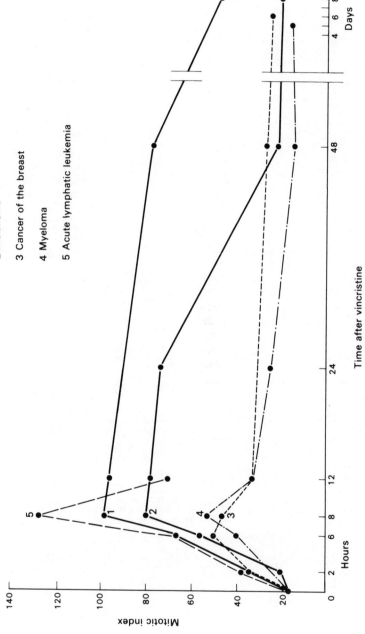

Fig. 6

Table 15. Results of chemotherapy in various oncological diseases.

EFFECT OF CHEMOTHERAPY	HAEMATOLOGIC MALIGNANCY	ADULT SOLID TUMOUR	PAEDIATRIC SOLID TUMOUR
Disease-free for long periods or cure	Acute lymphatic leukaemia, Stage III/IV Hodgkin's, Burkitt's tumour	Trophoblastic carcinoma, Testicular tumour	Wilm's, Ewing's sarcoma, Embryonal rhabdomyosarcoma, Retinoblastoma
Significant objective regression, Survival gain	Non-Hodgkin's lymphoma, Multiple myeloma, Chronic lymphatic leukaemia	Adenocarcinoma of breast, Adenocarcinoma of ovary	Neuroblastoma
Adjuvant chemotherapy		Breast adenocarcinoma, GI adenocarcinoma	Osteosarcoma
Transient response		Malignant melanoma, Soft tissue sarcoma, GI adenocarcinoma, Squamous carcinoma head and neck, Bronchial, Thyroid, Prostate bladder	

Vincristine is also known to increase the mitotic index. (Fig. 6)

The ideal chemotherapeutic agent should be capable of transportation to target cells, resist degradation on the way, attack a specific cell, be able to cross the cell membrane, and kill that cell.

It is now established that surgery, radiotherapy and chemotherapy in oncological diseases are effective either as single or combined agents. The primary tumour is surgically removed or destroyed by radiotherapy, hopefully before the disease has disseminated, but this is often not the case; chemotherapy used to control disseminated disease offers the best hope for reducing mortality in a number of different cancers. Modern chemotherapy can be curative or palliative to varying degrees depending on the type of cancer as indicated in Table 15.

CONCLUSION

Cancer chemotherapy has had a slow painstaking evolution, but until recently never fulfilling that ultimate aim of total cure. However, with the advent of combining drugs with no increase in toxicity, there have been dramatic improvements in certain diseases; the introduction of prophylactic therapy has also added a new but perhaps controversial dimension.

New drugs, such as, Adriamycin, Bleomycin, on their own have brought their particular advantage, and in combination are offering a better span of life to many previously resistant tumours. Amongst the most recent evaluated agents there may be the ideal drug, but it would appear that the biochemical facet for potential survival of most cancer,cells cannot be fully eradicated unless they exist microscopically; or a drug is developed which is purely specific against a particular tumour and its proliferating cells.

DISCUSSION

Question 1.   Since chemotherapy must be planned for the longer term, what facilities would Dr. Hanham advise for such extensive observation?   Do we require more resident facilities for these patients?

Answer.   A considerable burden is to be placed on all medical and paramedical services if many patients are to have prolonged chemotherapy, and it is developing into an integral part of cancer treatment.   Hopefully this can be carried out on an intermittent out-patient basis, although day care facilities would reduce the morbidity of treatment.

Question 2.   The American and Japanese pharmacologists have found that some types of orchids (Dendrobuin) are antibacterial and antitumour when used.   The Chinese also have some herbal cure for cancer.   Is there any truth in this and is there any research done on herbal cure?

Answer.   Many plant alkaloids have a pharmacological action, and some are used extensively in cancer treatment. The historical use of pharmacological compounds made from herbs is as old as civilisation, and some of these have a cytotoxic effect.   Their sophisticated clinical use is a much more recent development.

Question 3.   How can the newer chemotherapy be made more available on a national scale?

Answer.   Newer drugs used to-day can be very expensive. A recent costing showed that a patient with osteosarcoma, treated prophylactically with methotrexate for one year, amounted to £6,000.

New chemicals are also expensive to develop and their clinical use must be justified by clinical trials and the absence of toxicity.

Question 4.   Many patients are now being treated by chemotherapy.   At what point in this treatment is it possible for the general practitioner to take over the care of the patient?

Answer.   The complexities of chemotherapy are now so

considerable that there cannot be a point when the general
practitioner can assume overall care in the patient's
management.   Many complex regimes have been worked out,
particularly in relation to cell cycling, as already
described, or in prophylactic treatment, such as with
osteosarcoma.   The general practitioner cannot actively
participate in this, except to be aware of the complications
that can arise from these treatments, which continue
intermittently for many months or even years.   They must be
made aware of these side effects and be able to sustain the
patient through prolonged therapy.

COMBINATION TREATMENT

Michael Baum

Senior Lecturer and Honorary Consultant Surgeon
University Department of Surgery
Welsh National School of Medicine

INTRODUCTION

The mortality from the common cancers affecting the population of this country have remained disturbingly constant over recent years. (Table 1)   Furthermore, survival rates after 'curative' surgery in those patients treated in an apparently early stage leave little room for complacency. (Fig. 1)   Indeed, the small changes in cancer statistics reported over the last 50 years could equally well be ascribed to changes in population characteristics, changes in the techniques of data collection, or changes in the natural behaviour of the cancers, rather than to any real advances in treatment.

This may sound a rather gloomy start to a paper, but a critical appreciation of these facts has been the essential platform upon which an important "breakthrough" in our thinking concerning the management of solid tumours has taken place.   It is on the basis of this change in philosophy concerning the nature of the common cancers affecting man that the principles of combination therapy have been evolved.

TRADITIONAL VIEW OF THE MECHANISM OF SPREAD OF CANCER

Until the end of the last century little attempt was made at curative surgery for cancer.   This was mainly due to the appalling mortality resulting from major surgery at

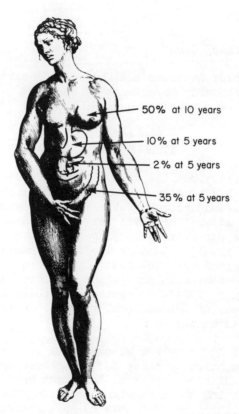

Figure 1.   Survival following "curative" treatment
            of common cancers

Table 1.   Mortality from common cancers in Wales.

				Year		
Site	Sex	1968	1969	1970	1971	1972
Stomach	M	485	562	557	500	531
	F	413	379	394	376	397
Colon and Rectum	M	418	426	427	440	462
	F	474	485	501	469	513
Bronchus	M	1106	1216	1184	1251	1296
	F	193	202	206	212	203
Breast	F	545	591	588	654	585

Report of the Chief Medical Officer.   Welsh Office 1974
                                                    H.M.S.O.

that time and the natural reluctance of the population to
submit themselves to such risks.   However, by the early
1900's most surgical techniques had been mastered,
anaesthesia was widely available and the principle of
asepsis was soundly established.   Alongside these
developments surgeons and pathologists described a concept
of behaviour of cancers upon which they designed the
operations for the eradication of the disease. (1)It was
taught that the cancer was an autonomous growth, that
spread in columns of cells from the organ of origin along
lymphatic channels, (small vessels that drain tissue fluid,)
until becoming arrested in the first set of lymph nodes
they met.   These nodes were thought to act as inert filter
traps, which collected the cancer cells, forming a secondary
or metastatic deposit.   With further passage of time the
malignant cells were released into the more distant lymph
channels with a further period of arrest at the next set of
lymph nodes.   And so the tumour was thought to progress
step by step until it reached the vital organs and became
incurable.   Developing out of this concept, the principle
of 'radical en bloc' surgery evolved.   The operations were

designed, not only to include the organ of origin of the
cancer, but as many groups of surrounding lymph nodes as was
compatible with the survival of the patient.   Furthermore,
the dissections were designed not to cut across any lymphatic
channels and so risk spilling cancer cells into the 'clean'
operative field.   As anaesthesia improved and blood
transfusions became available, surgeons extended the field
of surgery wider and, with the introduction of radiotherapy,
an attempt was made to 'sterilize' lymph nodes at the
periphery of the operative field or to mop up cancer cells
accidently spilled during surgery.   Such an approach would
have seemed eminently appropriate, say in 1910, but
developments in our knowledge of tumour biology over the
last 50 years has led to a critical re-appraisal of our
therapeutic approach.

MODERN CONCEPTS OF THE SPREAD OF CANCER
AND BIOLOGICAL PREDETERMINISM

Recent developments in the pathological sciences have
in the most part rendered the doctrines of the early decades
of the 20th century obsolete.   Cancer cells do not grow in
columns along the lymph channels, but embolize as single
cells or small clumps.   Most cancers invade the blood stream
directly, or enter the circulation via lymphatic/venous
communications.   Cancer cells may bypass or traverse lymph
nodes which, therefore, do not act as efficient filters.
For these reasons cancer cells may reach the vital organs,
such as, the brain, liver, or lungs, at an early stage and
even before the lymph nodes are obviously overwhelmed.
Furthermore, these lymph nodes, long thought to be inert,
are in fact a hostile soil for malignant seeds which can be
actively destroyed by the cells of natural defence
(lymphocytes and macrophages), which concentrate at these
sites.   And finally, to complicate the equation further,
the lymphocytes and macrophages do not merely act in passive
defence, but are thought also to have a limited capacity to
seek out and destroy the cancer cells shed into the general
circulation.

In the early 1950's the theory of biological
predeterminism was described.(2) It was suggested that the
outcome of treatment was decided, not by the extent of local
surgery and radiotherapy, but by the degree of blood-borne

undetected cancer cells (micrometastases) at the time of presentation, and that this was predetermined by the biological characteristics of that cancer.   Thus an unfavourable cancer with early spread by the general circulation would be incurable by the time it reached diagnosable proportions, whilst a favourable cancer with little potential for dissemination by the blood stream might remain curable by local treatment long after it had reached a detectable size.   Added to this are the recent advances in the science of tumour immunology (the natural resistance to cancer). (3)   We now regard the successful establishment of a focus of cancer in a regional lymph node, not as an inevitable sequence of the passage of time, but as the stigma of a lost battle between the cancer cell and nature's defences.

An acceptance of these newer concepts readily explains the facts about cancers, which clinicians face in their everyday struggle against the disease.   Firstly, wider fields of local treatment have not produced a greater number of cures because of the predetermined outcome of a cancer at presentation.   Secondly, patients whose lymph nodes are found to be replaced by cancer have such a bad prognosis that the majority have to be considered incurable by conventional therapy.   In such cases the involved node merely acts as an index of the certain existence of micrometastases throughout the body.

A most important clinical trial concerning the treatment of early breast cancer supports these latter assertions. (4)   The King's/Cambridge group compared simple mastectomy (removal of the breast alone) with simple mastectomy followed by regional radiotherapy (a radical approach aimed at sterilizing the operative field and all groups of lymph nodes surrounding the breast).   At 5 years after treatment there was absolutely no difference in survival between the patients treated by either of these two widely differing approaches.

ADJUVANT SYSTEMIC THERAPY

From the preceding discussion, it is apparent that to achieve a greater number of cures, beyond those cancers in the biologically favourable group, (i.e., non-metastasising or late metastasising,) some form of additive treatment designed to destroy the malignant cells that have reached the vital organs prior to diagnosis is essential.   The objectives of the local treatment are then re-defined in terms of local control for symptomatic relief.

For the rest of the discussion in this paper I wish to confine myself to carcinoma of the breast, which is the disease which lends itself best to study because of its superficial nature and because it is the disease where we have most experience in the use of adjuvant therapy. However, it is important to remember from the outset that in two respects breast cancer is somewhat atypical. Firstly, it is a tumour with a very prolonged latency with recurrences appearing up to twenty years after successful control of the local disease, and, secondly, it is a tumour known to be in part dependent on the hormone levels in the blood and as such can occasionally be influenced by endocrine manipulation.

The types of adjuvant systemic therapy that are available for carcinoma of the breast are as follows:

1.   Endocrine therapy

2.   Cytotoxic cancer chemotherapy

3.   Immunotherapy

1.   Endocrine Therapy

Endocrine therapy can be considered as either additive or ablative.   For reasons that are not yet well understood, some breast cancers respond if the patient is treated with oestrogens, androgens, progesterones or cortico-steroids. At the same time breast cancers also respond to the ablative operations, such as, oophorectomy, adrenalectomy or hypophysectomy.   None of these additive or ablative treatments are without unpleasant side effects.   Oestrogens can produce nausea, heart failure and cerebral vascular problems.   Androgens can produce virilization, hoarseness of the voice and hirsutism.   The cortico-steroids have their own catalogue of unpleasant side effects as well. Oophorectomy, although a very simple operative procedure, may produce acute menopausal symptoms and a psychological

blow to a woman who already has her fair share of problems.
Bilateral adrenalectomy is a major abdominal operation with
associated morbidity and the patients have to be maintained
thereafter on cortisone.   Hypophysectomy is also a major
and potentially hazardous operation and the patients have to
be maintained on a number of additive hormones to compensate
for the loss of endocrine control by the pituitary gland.

2.   Cytotoxic Cancer Chemotherapy

One of the most exciting developments in the treatment
of cancer over the last five to ten years has been the
discovery and synthesis of a wide variety of active chemical
agents which have the property of killing cancer cells at
doses which are reasonably well tolerated by normal tissues.
Furthermore, it has been discovered that the use of a number
of these drugs in combination has a synergistic tumorocidal
effect without additive toxicity.   The use of such drugs in
the treatment of the leukaemias and Hodgkin's disease has
produced the most impressive improvements in survival rates
for these otherwise fatal conditions.   In the management of
advanced breast cancer, combinations of these anti-cancer
drugs have produced worthwhile regressions with good palliation
that may last for up to two years in a patient who would
otherwise be condemned to a certain death within a few months.
Unfortunately, for these drugs to be effective, it seems
inevitable that there should be some unwelcome side effects
as well.   Thus the most effective combinations of drugs all
produce alopecia and bone marrow suppression with the risks
of anaemia and overwhelming infections.   Most of the drugs
produce nausea, vomiting and disturbances in bowel action as
well.   Finally, it is not known what the long term effects
of such potent agents are likely to be as, until now, they
have only been used in patients with a short expectation of
life.

3.   Immunotherapy

As described earlier, there are natural defence
mechanisms in the body that can deal with small numbers of
malignant cells and perhaps even prevent the development of
cancers in the first instance.   It would seem logical,
therefore, to attempt to stimulate these natural mechanisms

to overcome the tumour burden remaining after successful
clearance of the primary tumour.   There are two approaches
to this problem - specific and non-specific immunotherapy.
Specific immunotherapy is designed to stimulate the patient's
lymphocytes to recognize the specific antigens (the abnormal
surface characteristics) of the tumour cell.   This could be
achieved by innoculating the patient at various sites of the
body with either killed cancer cells from their own tumours,
or else antigen-rich fragments of their own tumours.   The
second approach, known as non-specific immunotherapy, is
thought to work by the stimulation of the macrophages rather
than the lymphocytes.   These cells are responsible for
ingesting and processing the antigen before handing it over
to the lymphocyte and, in addition, when activated, they have
the unique property of being able to recognize cancer cells
and destroy them on surface contact.   Non-specific
immunotherapy can be achieved by injecting live or dead
bacterial products and the two agents widely in use at
present are B.C.G. (the variety of tubercule bacillus which
is used for immunization against tuberculosis) and
Corynebacterium Parvum which is a bacterium which does not
normally produce infections in man, but has the peculiar
property of being a very potent immuno-stimulant.

      Unfortunately, we do not fully understand yet the
mechanisms of immunity to cancer.   There are even some
theoretical objections to the use of immunotherapy in
patients.   Under certain experimental circumstances, the
tumour can actually be enhanced by inappropriate meddling
with the control mechanisms.   Apart from that, the bacterial
agents used for non-specific immunotherapy may themselves
produce infection, fever and malaise.

      For the many reasons enumerated above, one would
hesitate to prescribe any form of additive therapy to those
patients with a good prognosis, that is, patients where we
feel sure that cure has been achieved after local treatment
alone.   For this reason I wish to review the question of
prognostic indices which may enable us to select those
patients who are likely to die of their disease in spite of
successful local control.

PROGNOSTIC INDICES

Prognostic indices for breast cancer can be considered under four headings:

1. The Regional Lymph Nodes.

2. Radiological and Isotopic Indices of Dissemination.

3. Biochemical Indices of Dissemination.

4. Immunological Status.

1. The status of the regional lymph nodes, as studied by the pathologist after mastectomy, gives us the most certain information about the prognosis of a woman with apparently early breast cancer. Many studies have demonstrated unequivocally that the degree of malignant involvement of the regional lymph nodes correlates very closely with the chances of survival. (5) Thus, if none of the nodes examined contain malignant cells, then that woman probably has a 70% chance of cure by local treatment alone. Whereas, if more than four lymph nodes are involved with metastases, then there is almost no chance that that woman will be alive 10 years after mastectomy. It is interesting to note in passing that, if the lymph nodes are uninvolved with cancer but demonstrate microscopic evidence of reaction suggestive of an immune response, then these patients carry a better prognosis than might otherwise be expected. (6)

2. No patient should be subjected to mastectomy unless they have had some form of radiological survey of the skeleton and chest. Most clinicians would now agree that, if there are lung or skeletal metastases seen on X-rays, then these patients should not be subjected to an unnecessary operation. Over the last five or six years new radio-isotope techniques have been developed, which appear to be demonstrating skeletal metastases at a much earlier stage than conventional radiology. About 25% of patients with early breast cancer and normal skeletal X-rays have abnormal radio-isotope bone scans and most of these will develop overt skeletal metastases over the succeeding five years. (7) Unfortunately, these techniques need expensive equipment which is not always available, the results are only reliable in a few specialised centres and it is probably too early to suggest that bone scanning should be used on a wide scale for predicting prognosis.

3.   Biochemical indices of dissemination would be the ideal solution to the problem as a simple blood or urine test might give some index of vital organ involvement. Several centres now are analysing the blood and urine for abnormal products that suggest that the bone or liver is involved. (8, 9)   Results along these lines look promising but as yet there is no reliable tumour marker that gives more information than that obtained by a study of the regional lymph nodes.

4.   Following studies of tumour immunology in experimental animals in cancer research laboratories throught the world, there has been a vast expenditure of money and effort into studying the immunological status of patients with cancer in an attempt to develop useful prognostic indices.   It is true that an exhaustive immunological profile carried out on large numbers of women with breast cancer will show small differences in results between patients with advanced cancers and those with localised small cancers, but as far as predicting the outcome of treatment in women with early disease, the results have proved very disappointing and non-reproducable.

It would appear, therefore, pending on future developments, that the best prognostic index available in women being treated for breast cancer is the pathological status of the axillary lymph nodes (that is, the lymph nodes accessible in the armpit at the time of mastectomy,) and for this reason several clinical trials are progressing to evaluate additive systemic treatment in patients having mastectomies for breast cancer, who have lymph node involvement.

CURRENT STATUS OF CLINICAL TRIALS
FOR ADJUVANT CHEMOTHERAPY IN EARLY BREAST CANCER

There are a number of important clinical trials in progress for early breast cancer, comparing local therapy alone with local therapy plus additive cytotoxic chemotherapy in those patients with pathologically involved lymph nodes. Two important trials have recently been reported in the American literature. (10, 11)   Firstly, the American Co-operative Study Group (N.S.A.B.P.) have reported on the use of a single oral cytotoxic drug (Melphalan) in patients

undergoing radical mastectomy where one or more lymph nodes
have been found to be involved with tumour.   Although the
study has only been going about 2 years, a significant
benefit has been shown for the premenopausal women receiving
the additive cytotoxic agent.   Secondly, the Italian co-
operative group, with headquarters in Milan, have reported
on a study for women having radical mastectomy with
aggressive cytotoxic chemotherapy using a four-drug
combination for women with lymphatic involvement.   Again,
within a year or two of the study being started, a
significant benefit has been shown for the patients receiving
the additive treatment.   In this study there was no doubt
that the toxicity was quite significant but, as the authors
implied, it is better to be bald than dead.   Both these
studies use radical mastectomy as the primary local treatment.
Many workers in this field consider that radical surgery
(which involves removal of the muscles on the chest wall and
total clearance of axillary contents) is over-treatment.
Local control of the disease can equally well be achieved
by more conservative procedures.   For this reason, studies
in this country, by the King's/Cambridge group and the
Edinburgh group, are designed at looking at the effect of
additive cytotoxic therapy following conservative local
surgery where the axillary node status is ascertained by a
simple biopsy.   The results of these and other such trials
should be reported within the next few years.

CONCLUSION

     After about 50 years of frustration concerning the
diminishing returns of cancer surgery, there are at last
some genuine reasons for optimism.   There has been a major
breakthrough (dare I use that hackneyed expression) in the
treatment of solid tumours in man.   It is interesting to
reflect that this breakthrough has not been achieved by the
development of a new operation, nor largely due to the
development of a new drug, but really follows on a new
doctrine which more completely describes the behaviour of
cancer.   Clinicians must start thinking of cancer as a
generalized disease until proved otherwise and surgeons
must accept that their technical virtuosity alone cannot
defeat the subtle aggression of the microscopic cancer cell.

REFERENCES

1.   Halsted, W.S. 1907. The results of radical operations
       for the cure of cancer of the breast. Annals of
       Surgery 46:1.

2.   Macdonald, I. 1951. Biological predeterminism in human
       cancer. Surgery, Gynaecology and Obstetrics 92:443.

3.   Fisher, B. 1971. The present status of tumour immunology.
       Advances in Surgery, Volume 5. Welch, C.E. and
       Hardy, J.D., Editors. Year Book Medical Publishers,
       Chicago.

4.   Management of early cancer of the breast. Cancer Research
       Campaign Study. British Medical Journal. In Press.

5.   Fisher, B. 1970. The surgical dilemma in the primary
       therapy of invasive breast cancer: a critical
       appraisal. Current Problems in Surgery. Year Book
       Medical Publishers, Chicago.

6.   Black, M.M. and Speer, F.D. 1958. Sinus histiocytosis
       of lymph nodes in cancer. Surgery, Gynaecology and
       Obstetrics 106:163.

7.   Galasko, C.S.B. 1975. The significance of occult skeletal
       metastases detected by skeletal scintigraphy in
       patients with otherwise apparently early mammary
       cancer. British Journal of Surgery 62:694.

8.   Roberts, J.G., Keyser, J.W. and Baum, M. 1975. Serum
       alpha-1-acid glycoprotein as an index of
       dissemination in breast cancer. British Journal of
       Surgery 62:816.

9.   Roberts, J.G., Williams, M. and Baum, M. 1975. The
       prediction of bone involvement in breast cancer by
       the "hypronosticon" test. Clinical Oncology 1:33.

10. Fisher, B., Carbonne, P., Economou, S.G. et al. 1975.
       L-Phenylalanine Mustard (L-PAM) in the management
       of primary breast cancer. The New England Journal
       of Medicine 292:117.

11. Bonadonna, G., Brusamolino, E., Valagusso, P. et al.
       1976. Combination chemotherapy as an adjuvant
       treatment in operable breast cancer. The New
       England Journal of Medicine 294:405.

DISCUSSION

Question 1.   It seems that chemotherapy will play an
increasing part in breast carcinoma.   Does Mr. Baum regard
the testing of these chemicals against breast carcinoma in
tissue culture as important?   Are there facilities available
for these tests to be made?

Answer.   Tissue cultures assay for chemotherapy
planning have proved very disappointing, mainly because it
is almost impossible to persuade breast cancer to grow in
vitro.

Question 2.   Do cortico-steroids just increase a sense
of wellbeing in terminal cancer patients?

Answer.   No, they may produce undoubted reduction in
tumour bulk by interference with the endocrine control of
hormone-sensitive cancers or by the reduction of oedema
around cerebral or hepatic metastases.

Question 3.   Since combination treatment is now
vitally important for cancer patients, is there a uniform
system of joint clinics in operation in the United Kingdom?

Answer.   The simple answer is - No, there is not a
uniform system.   I would like to endorse heartily everything
Mr. Ian Burn said about the teamwork approach to this problem.
I still believe, like Mr. Ian Burn, that the clinician to
whom the patient is first referred, (in the case of the
common solid tumours this will always be the surgeon,) should
retain a responsibility for that patient until discharged as
cured or until his death.   At the same time the individual
clinician has to work in a team, and in Cardiff we have such
a team which has developed in the same way as at Charing Cross
and Westminster Hospitals, but unfortunately there is no
uniform pattern.   I hope the British Association of Surgical
Oncology will pioneer this type of development.

Question 4.   Does Mr. Baum see an increasing use for
pre-operative radiotherapy for cancer patients, and how does
this affect subsequent surgery?

Answer.   This is an interesting problem which it would
take a long time to answer.   In theory it is very attractive
because the cancer cells at the periphery of an operative

field are those best oxygenated and, therefore, most likely
to be sensitive to radiotherapy and at the same time most
likely to be left by the surgeon.   There are trials in
progress at present, run by the M.R.C., for pre-operative
radiotherapy for rectal cancer.   At the same time there
are problems from the surgeon's point of view.   The healing
of the wound after radiotherapy may be delayed and there is
the theoretical hazard associated with immuno-suppression
from regional radiotherapy, which may enhance tumour growth.

HOW TO PREVENT CANCER

Francis J.C. Roe

Independent Consultant in Experimental Pathology
and Cancer Research

This symposium is concerned exclusively with cancer.
Nevertheless, we need to view the subject of prevention in
the broader context of all causes of disease and death and,
indeed, of all the complex problems which fact the human
race.   In Table 1 is set out a personal appraisal of where
the prevention of cancer fits into the list of problems
which demand our most urgent attention.   Both the problems
and the solutions to them are interrelated: to succeed in
finding out how to prevent cancer without knowing how to
control population growth, prevent war, and to preserve the
environment from pollution, particularly by mutagens, would
be a hollow victory.

Table 1.   Problems facing mankind.

1.   Population control.

2.   Preservation of the environment.

3.   Prevention of war.

4.   Improvement of the quality of human life:

    (a) Food and shelter,

    (b) Prevention of disease, including cancer,

    (c) Personal freedom.

The existence of a problem does not dictate that there exists a solution to it. Thus it is by no means certain that all forms of cancer can be prevented, or that death from cancer can be entirely avoided. Indeed, it is debatable whether the total avoidance of death from cancer is an appropriate aim until we have squarely faced a problem which so far man, as a species, has not been prepared to face. If we knew how to prevent all deaths from cancer and heart disease, we would almost certainly be faced by an alarming increase in age-associated morbidity and in deaths attributable to age-associated diseases. Do we as a society want this? Are those of us who are able-bodied, able-minded and in the full cry of our working lives really prepared, as individuals, to take on the additional burden of caring for a greatly increased non-productive retired and aging population? Is the average quality of the dying process likely to be improved by abolishing cancer as a disease? The concept of the "quality of life" is widely held and debated. Personally, I am sure that we need also to consider the "quality of death." I am not an advocate of euthanasia, but I know of several old people who have out-lived their spouses and friends, whose senses are failing and who want to die. Our society is as yet a long way from knowing how to cherish its old people and make them feel wanted. Little would be gained by preventing people from dying of cancer if they then have to endure the agonies of rejection and neglect by the society in which they live.

In making these general remarks, I am not implying that cancerous diseases cannot and should not be prevented. On the contrary, I seek only to define more clearly what our aim should be. In so far as many factors, which predispose to cancers in man, have been positively identified, we already have some insight into how at least a proportion of cases of the disease could be prevented. An oft-quoted view is that 80% or more of all cancers are due to exposure to environmental factors rather than to genetic defects. This, of course, is over-simplistic because genetic and environmental factors tend to interact in the causation of disease. Nor does it really set the target of cancers which we should expect to be able to prevent at 80%. The figure of 80% is arrived at by comparing death rates from different forms of cancer in various countries and assuming that rates in excess of the lowest rates are due to avoidable environmental factors. The justification for making the

latter assumption is to some extent supported by studies
showing changes in death rates from particular types of
cancer in people who migrate from one environment to another
and in their children and children's children.   On the
other hand, it should not be forgotten that environments
which are associated with low rates of death from some forms
of cancer tend to be associated with high rates of death for
other forms of the disease. (Table 2)   It would not be
possible on the basis of presently available knowledge to
define an environment in which humans could really expect to
experience only 20% of the present risk of death from all
forms of cancer.

Table 2.   Age-adjusted death rates from cancers in males in
           4 different countries in 1964-5 (from Segi et al,
                                                        1969).

	E & W	US White	Japan	France
Mouth	3	4	1	9
Larynx	2	2	2	10
Lung	68	37	13	26
Stomach	23	9	69	21
Intestine (except rectum)	12	14	3	12
Liver etc.	3	5	15	9
Urinary tract	7	5	2	5
Prostate	12	13	2	14
ALL SITES	180	144	140	169

Cancer is not a single disease but a broad group of diseases with different causes and different manifestations. Some types are associated with a variety of causative factors and some causative factors are associated with increased risk of more than one type of the disease.   For most forms of cancer, except those peculiar to childhood, the risk of development increases logarithmically with age.   It is thought by some that the increase with age is indicative of increasing susceptibility of aging cells and tissues to undergo a cancerous change on exposure to an environmental carcinogen.   The results of a recent study in mice (Peto et al, 1975), however, were inconsistent with this explanation. We showed that the risk of developing skin tumours in response to the repeated application of a carcinogen (3,4-benzpyrene) to the skin varied directly with the period since the start of exposure irrespective of the age at which exposure started. (Fig. 1)

This is, in fact, a very encouraging finding because it means that reducing the exposure of people while they are still young is likely to bring down, perhaps substantially, their subsequent risk of developing cancer.   If we had found that mice grew progressively more susceptible to the effects of benzpyrene as they grew older, then the most one could have reasonably hoped from reducing exposure to carcinogens is a relatively short postponement of age at death from cancer.

This, conveniently, brings me back to what it is reasonable to hope can be done in relation to the prevention of cancer.   Cancerous diseases are a feature not only of man but of all vertebrate species.   Increasing incidence rates with age is the rule for most of these diseases in most species.   This suggests that genetic and environmental factors which predispose to cancers are widespread and that cancerous diseases are indeed a part of nature and not something superimposed on nature by man.   Common sense, if nothing else, therefore, suggests that it is probably unrealistic to hope to prevent all forms of cancer.   All we may reasonably hope to do is, by genetic counselling and reducing exposure to known potent carcinogens, to push cancer incidence curves somewhat to the right – so that cancer competes more fairly with other causes of death in the elderly and less often cuts people off in their prime or early retirement.

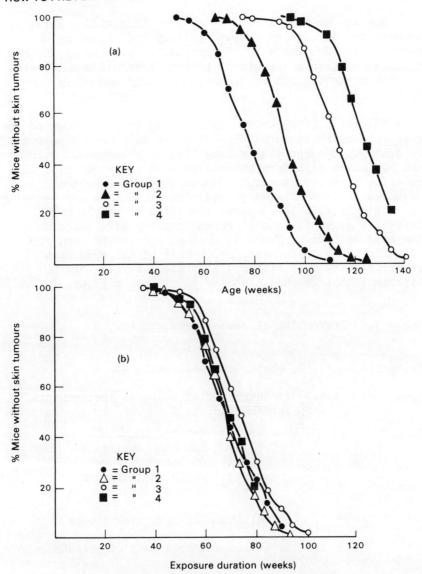

Figure 1.   Development of skin tumours in four groups of mice
             in response to 3,4-benzpyrene applied to the skin
             from the ages of 10 (Group 1), 25 (Group2), 40
             (Group 3) and 55 weeks (Group 4).   After allowing
             for deaths from non-specific causes, risk of tumour
             development was found to depend entirely on exposure
             duration (b) and not at all on age (a) (from Peto
             et al., 1975).

How are we most likely to achieve this aim?   Firstly, we need to distinguish between primary and secondary prevention. (See Table 3)   I propose to confine my further remarks to certain aspects of primary prevention and leave to others the big and important subject of secondary prevention.

Mulvihill (1975) recently reviewed what is known of the role of genetic factors in relation to malignant diseases. He draws up a surprisingly long list of chromosomal disorders and Mendelian disorders associated with increased risk of specific forms of cancer.   One unfortunate aspect of advances in other fields of medicine is that we are becoming increasingly able to preserve the lives of people with defective genes to ages at which they may have children with the same defects.   There is thus an increasing need for effective genetic counselling.   Most of the syndromes referred to by Mulvihill are at present rare.   It is important that we should strive to make them rarer.

Table 3.   Prevention of deaths from cancer.

Primary: 1.   Genetic counselling.

                  2.   Avoidance of exposure to environmental
                       carcinogens:

                            (i)   Natural chemicals
                            (ii)   Man-made chemicals
                            (iii) Oncogenic viruses
                            (iv)   Ionising radiation
                            (v)   Hormone disturbances

Secondary: 1.   Surveillance of high risk groups.

                  2.   Detection and treatment of precancerous
                       states.

                  3.   Early diagnosis.

                  4.   More effective treatment of established
                       disease.

It is widely believed that the only important
environmental carcinogens are man-made chemicals and that
cancer is man's punishment for interfering with nature.   I
am not sure whether Adam was responsible for the upkeep of
the Garden of Eden but, if he was, then every time he dug up
a weed he could be said to have been interfering with nature.
Likewise Eve should obviously have waited until that apple
dropped.   Or have I got it wrong?   Is man, as a part of
nature behaving naturally when he tills the soil and picks
the fruit before it falls and bruises, or is consumed by
birds, or wasps, or is fermented by micro-organisms?   What
I am trying to say is that it is very difficult to draw the
line between the intelligent but natural exploitation of
nature by man and undesirable interference by man with the
process of nature.

At the recent meeting on the Detection and Prevention
of Cancer in New York, Dr. Ernest Wynder, well-known for his
research on the role of smoking in relation to lung cancer,
expressed the opinion that carcinogens in food are almost
certainly responsible for far more cancers than smoking or
industrial chemicals combined.   Apart from the chemicals
which are deliberately added to food-stuffs during processing
or which contaminate them (e.g. pesticide residues,
atmospheric fall-out), we have to remember that foodstuffs
themselves may be carcinogenic, or may be contaminated with
naturally-occurring carcinogens.   Governments and
international agencies, such as, the World Health Organisation
and Food and Agricultural Organisation, keep a very careful
watch on the safety of chemicals which are added to food, or
which may contaminate it.   Hitherto much less attention has
been paid to the safety of foodstuffs themselves and to
searching for yet more naturally-occurring carcinogens
which may contaminate food.   Studies in laboratory animals
show unequivocally that over-eating itself may greatly
increase cancer risk.   So far, it is not clear whether the
same is true for humans.

There are serious difficulties in relating consumption
of food chemicals thought to be carcinogenic on the basis of
laboratory tests to cancer incidence in humans.   Thus, it
is not yet absolutely certain that any of the naturally
occurring carcinogens shown in Table 4 cause cancer in man.
However, there is now very strong circumstantial evidence
that aflatoxin is mainly responsible for the very high

Table 4.   Some natural carcinogens.

<u>Mycotoxins</u>:

        Aflatoxin

        Sterigmatocystin

        Islanditoxin

        Luteoskyrin

        Cyclochlorotin

<u>Plant components</u>:

        Cycasin

        Certain pyrrolizidine alkaloids

        Safrole

        Certain anti-thyroid substances

        ? Plant components with oestrogenic
                             activity

        A constituent of bracken fern

<u>Nitrosamines</u> formed by the consumption of food
             containing secondary or tertiary
             amines and food (e.g. spinach) or
             drinking water containing nitrite.

incidence of liver cancer in certain parts of Africa.

    In the field of man-made chemicals added to food,
there continues to be deep concern about the possible dangers
of using nitrite as a preservative for meat and also as a
fertilizer of soil.   There now exists a large number of
reports of the formation of carcinogenic nitrosamines in the
stomach following the simultaneous ingestion of food or drugs
containing secondary or tertiary amines and nitrite, which
is present in drinking water, natural foodstuffs, such as,

spinach, and preserved meats, etc.   In laboratory animals
it is possible to produce cancers in animals by the
simultaneous oral administration of nitrite and secondary
amines.   Personally, I believe there is reason to be
seriously concerned about possible cancer hazard from
nitrosamines formed in this way.   On the other hand, as I
shall explain, the problem poses a dilemma which at present
has no easy or obvious solution.

I am far less certain whether some of the other cancer
scares which have hit the newspaper headlines during recent
years merit serious attention.   In the United States, there
is an ever-increasing list of banned chemicals (including
cyclamates, DDT, dieldrin, heptachlor, Myrex) for which there
is no substantial evidence of cancer hazard for man and, in
some cases, persuasive evidence of safety for man.   On the
one hand, it is encouraging for those dedicated to the
primary prevention of cancer that research resources are at
long last being used to investigate the carcinogenic
potential of ordinary chemicals.   On the other hand, it is,
in the long-run, probably not necessarily sensible to ban
widely used chemicals on grounds of mere suspicion, or
inadequate evidence of likely hazard.   It is certain that
an environment entirely free of carcinogens cannot be created.
Man, like his forbears in the evolutionary tree, has to be
content to live in a sea of carcinogens.   It is conceivable
that by using one chemical that is very weakly carcinogenic
he can protect himself against exposure from a much more
potent carcinogen, or against the risk of acute death from
infection or poisoning.   This is illustrated by the dilemma
referred to above concerning the use of nitrite as a meat
preservative.   Its use constitutes the main protection
against a serious and commonly fatal form of food poisoning,
botulism.   In the presence of nitrite the bacterium which
produces the toxin cannot grow.   If we abandon the use of
nitrite as a preservative of cooked meats, the risk of
botulism is liable to increase.

During the next few years we will have to face many
other real dilemmas in relation to cancer.   Firstly,
evidence is beginning to emerge that the risk of liver tumour
development in women taking the contraceptive pill is not as
negligible as has hitherto been believed.   Indeed, some
fear that we might be on the threshold of a serious epidemic
of this kind of cancer due to the pill.   Secondly, it is

becoming ever clearer that the cancer hazard from exposure
to asbestos dust is increasing.   If we abandon the use of
the contraceptive pill we are bound to magnify the problem
of population control.   If we abandon the use of asbestos,
we will have to face increased risks of fire and a multitude
of problems in relation to manufacturing processes and
building construction.   It is essential that very careful
risk/benefit evaluations are made before the use of such
chemicals is banned.   In the long-run it is also vitally
important that such decisions are made not solely in the
context of cancer control, but in the broader context of the
problems listed in Table 1.

        Twenty years or so ago cancer prevention was hardly on
the map as a subject.   Chemicals that cause cancer were
being experimented with in laboratories, and reports of studies
on laboratory rats and mice filled the cancer journals, but
many of the chemicals used in these studies are not present
in the human environment and the relevance of many of the
laboratory studies to the possibilities of preventing cancer
in man was not immediately obvious.   During the past two
decades the situation has completely changed.   Governments
and other institutions have become aware of the fact that
"Prevention is indeed better than cure."   Scientists have
discovered chemical carcinogens that are really likely to be
relevant to the causation of cancer in humans.   A prolonged
period of freedom from world war has enabled epidemiologists
to relate cancer risk to exposure to specific environmental
agents.   The development of computers has facilitated the
investigation of complex problems that could not previously
have been tackled.   During the last few years the possibility
of health hazard from exposure to chemicals at work has at
last come to be taken seriously in the USA, the UK and other
countries.   At the same time far more people have been made
aware of the importance of conservation and of the dangers of
pollution.

        I am, of course, delighted with these developments, but
at the same time I am uneasy lest the pendulum should swing
too far - lest those dedicated to the abolition of cancer
risk should seek to ban important chemicals and thereby throw
men out of work, and alter the whole fabric of society, on the
basis of no more than suspicion of cancer hazard and without
a careful, in-depth evaluation of the risks and benefits
associated with the proposed ban.

REFERENCES

Mulvihill, J.J. 1975. "Congenital and genetic diseases" in
    "Persons at High Risk of Cancer," edited by J.F.
    Fraumeni. Academic Press, New York, pp. 3-35.

Peto, R., Roe, F.J.C., Lee, P.N., Levy, L. and Clack, J.
    1975. "Cancer and Aging in Mice and Men," Brit. J.
    Cancer 32:411.

Segi, M., Kurihara, M. and Matsuyama, T. 1969. "Cancer
    Mortality for Selected Sites in 24 Countries," published
    by the Dept. of Public Health, Tohoku University School
    of Medicine, Sendai, Japan.

DISCUSSION

Question 1.   Could the speaker please outline the
dangers to health of the use of "Blue" and "White" asbestos,
how widespread they are and precautions that can be taken
both by workers with asbestos and the general public?

Since we have known for several years about the serious
risk from asbestos, was this knowledge made widely known and
positive action taken against this risk?

Answer.   It has long been recognised that the inhalation
of asbestos dust is dangerous.   The dust particles are long
and thin, (i.e., fibrous,) and tend to be carried in the
airstream during breathing into the deepest parts of the lung.
There they lodge and, partly because of their shape, size and
insolubility, the body finds it difficult to get rid of them.
Phagocytic cells, which try to remove them, die in the process
and their accumulation and death is followed by the development
of scar tissue.   This briefly is the explanation of the
disease, asbestosis.   Exactly why cancers of the lung itself
and of the membrane covering the lung, the pleura, arise, is
not known.   Certainly these diseases are associated with the
presence in the lung and pleura of persisting asbestos fibres,
but whether the cancers arise non-specifically from scar
tissue or are due to carcinogens being liberated slowly over
long periods from the fibres is a mystery.   Apart from cancers
of the lung and pleura, the inhalation of asbestos dust also
predisposes to cancers of the membranes covering abdominal
organs, the peritoneum.   Whether persons exposed to asbestos
dust are at increased risk of developing cancer of the

gastro-intestinal tract, (e.g., stomach, colon,) which has been claimed, is not certain.

Several types of asbestos are used commercially. They differ in several ways and particularly in colour and fibre shape. The long, strong, thin blue fibres of crocidolite asbestos seem to be the most dangerous. Chrysotile (white) asbestos fibres seem to be less dangerous.

Although the risks of asbestosis and cancer have long been recognised, it has only become apparent recently that precautions necessary to control the risk of asbestosis are not adequate to eliminate the risk of cancer. This is particularly clear in the case of cancers of the pleura and peritoneum (mesotheliomas) of which asbestos exposure seems to be virtually the only cause. Because smoking is also associated with lung cancer, it is difficult to be sure to what extent asbestos exposure is currently increasing the incidence of this disease. There are presently occurring up to 200 new cases of mesothelioma a year in this country. Obviously no one can be satisfied that precautions are adequate. Exposure is clearly much more dangerous than was at one time supposed. The use of blue asbestos has been largely abandoned for many purposes in favour of the less hazardous white forms of asbestos, especially chrysotile. However, demolition workers, ship-breakers and others may still be exposed to blue asbestos dust, especially when they come to dismantling heat or fire insulation systems. In any case, the extent to which white asbestos dust may be inhaled without real danger is not yet really clear. It would be wise to assume that no level of exposure to any form of asbestos dust is really safe and that stringent precautions are needed against such exposure. There is no evidence that asbestos in non-inhalable forms - e.g., asbestos sheeting - constitutes a hazard.

Question 2. Would Dr. Roe give his assessment of the contribution made to potential colonic cancer prevention by the dietary theories of Cleave, Burkitt, Trowell, et al? Mr. Burkitt and others have recommended a high fibre diet in which food passes through the intestine and reaches the anus much more quickly than it does in the case of the diet eaten normally in this country.

Answer. This is a theory which still needs to be

tested.   It has been developed by a very intelligent
interpretation of what Dr. Burkitt has seen.   A controlled
trial of people in this country eating two different sorts
of diet - a costly and time-consuming prospective study -
this scientific study is now needed.   I am quite sure that,
if people in this country adopted the sort of foods that
Africans eat, which pass through the gastro-intestinal tract
more quickly than the foods we eat in this country, we would
see changes in the incidence of some types of cancer, -
in fact, a lowering of the incidence of some forms of cancer
and possibly a raising of the incidence of other forms of
cancer.

Question 3.   In view of the great risk from radioactivity is Dr. Roe satisfied regarding the monitoring of
radiation in the atmosphere and precautions against possible
plutonium disaster?

Answer.   In the real world, some level of exposure to
hazard has to be accepted.   This is true for cancer of the
skin due to the sun's rays.   It is probably true for cancer
risk from asbestos dust and it is certainly true for cancer
risk from ionizing radiation.   In the context of all the
other dangers which threaten life, it is probably fair to say
that adequate attention has been and is being paid to the
monitoring of the atmosphere for radioactivity and to the
formulation of precautions against disasters from plutonium
and other sources of ionizing radiation.

Question 4.   How important is subnormal health for the
development of a malignant disease?

Answer.   This is a complex question.   Some agents
which cause cancer, also cause ill health;   for instance,
asbestos gradually destroys the lungs and then goes on to
cause cancers of the lungs and pleura.   Cancers very often
arise in diseased tissues or organs, but often the extent of
the disease is insufficient to cause a noticeable
deterioration in health, so that the first sign of disease
is the onset of cancer.   Emotional problems are associated
with changes in hormonal status.   There is some evidence
that such changes may favour malignant growth.   There are,
however, many forms of subnormal health, both physical and
mental, in which there is no excess of cancer risk.

ORGANISING CANCER WORK

Ian Burn

Consultant Surgeon and Surgical Oncologist

Charing Cross Hospital, London

The magnitude of the problem is best illustrated by
some figures.   In 1970, there were 154,351 registered new
cases of cancer in England and Wales, and 115,729 deaths
were reported.   There is every reason to suppose that in
most areas of malignant disease the incidence is increasing,
so it may be assumed that by 1980, in a few years time,
there will be about 175,000 new cases of cancer a year in
England and Wales.   Most malignant diseases are treated in
hospitals, at least in the first instance, and the number of
hospital beds occupied at any one time by patients with
cancer is considerable, probably representing about 10 per
cent of the whole.   The length of stay of a cancer patient
varies considerably, but may be prolonged.   Hospital
resources, consultative, investigative and therapeutic, are
frequently required by patients on a continuing basis after
a period of in-patient care.   Many patients will die, but
others will continue to be kept under regular follow-up,
with a cumulative work load.   The family doctor sees
relatively few new patients with cancer each year, ten on
the average.   Like the hospital, however, the requirements
of previously treated patients are such that the family
doctor's work load is also cumulative, embracing his role of
counselling, prescribing for and rehabilitating the surviving
patient, and providing all the necessary support for the
patients dying from the disease and for their relatives.

As well as these clinical aspects of cancer, there are
two other vital components to be considered, namely
educational and research.   The former involves both the
public and the caring professions.   Such effort as has been

247

made in the past to define and practice cancer education
has been limited, both by the absence of any concerted plan
of campaign and the facilities to put theory into practice.

Cancer research is familiar to us all.   The slogans
and appeals have been with us for decades, but what are the
realities of the situation.   Until recently, clinicians in
the United Kingdom participated in only a very minor way in
fundamental research.   Modifications and development of
surgical and radiotherapeutic techniques took place during
the early decades of the century and record-keeping became
more proficient in the hands of interested clinicians.
Laboratory cancer research scientists worked in a vacuum,
however, and their activities were confined almost entirely
to work with small animals.   This has now changed
dramatically, with an explosion of activity which is filling
the journals.   There is growing co-operation between
scientist and clinician, and much of the activity now
centres around the study of human tumours and patients with
malignant diseases.   This development is perhaps the most
encouraging of all aspects of cancer work, and all that
would seem to be lacking now (apart from money) is an
overall plan of organisation.   Maybe this is not really
required, and cancer research should be allowed to flourish
on an individual basis.   There would seem to be some sense,
however, in at least providing the means for dissemination
of the wealth of ideas and information that exists on the
subject now, and for ensuring that facilities for research
are equally and sensibly distributed.

These then are the three areas for consideration.   The
clinical practice of treating malignant diseases, education
both of the public and caring professions, and cancer
research.   These are vast requirements, and, as if to
provide a timely recognition of this, a new word has
appeared on the medical scene in the United Kingdom, which
has the virtue of embracing all aspects of cancer work -
ONCOLOGY.   Used extensively in Europe, and latterly in the
Americas, the term was slow in being adopted here, but has
now arrived.   Earlier objections to the word have largely
disappeared and it is rapidly achieving common usage in
medical practice.   Whatever one may think about its
derivation and sonic value, it does provide an international
generic term which is understood by all working in the field.
No doubt in time the public will also become familiar with

it, and it is possible that by lessening the use of the
word <u>cancer</u> it may reduce the emotive associations of
malignant disease.

ONCOLOGICAL CENTRES

The need for organising cancer work was recognised by
the Department of Health some years ago, resulting in the
establishment of the four major "Oncological Centres," in
Leeds, Manchester, Southampton and Surrey.   These four
centres are evolving in their own separate ways.   While
some are at a more advanced stage of evolution than others,
they all appear to be achieving the original intent of
combining specialist medical care of patients with
educational and research needs in the regions concerned.
This is very creditable and there is no doubt that the
experiment of defining and supporting these four centres
has been fully justified.   Whether further similar centres
should be created and supported is debatable, however, and
decisions on this must await the careful evaluation of those
already established.   In fact, the national needs may be
better served in other ways, and it is useful to consider
what might be done.

ONCOLOGISTS

On the professional side, the specialty of radiotherapy
has matured over the years, and this form of treatment has
now an established and vital role in the management of
malignant diseases.   A body of specialists staff the
various radiotherapy departments throughout the country,
and they have a total commitment to the problem.   Their
departments have formed the focal points in hospitals for
concentrated effort in cancer, and, where joint tumour
clinics have been formed, they have centred around the
radiotherapists.

Surgeons and physicians have been dilatory in
recognising the special needs of treating cancer.   In the
case of the physicians, this has been through force of
circumstances, in that, until the advent of cytotoxic
chemotherapy, there was little, if any, scope for medicinal
treatment of cancer.   The surgeons have no such excuse and

it is regrettable that to date no plans have yet emerged for
defining the surgeon's role in the future management of
malignant diseases.   There has been a natural evolvement of
certain specialist clinics dealing, for example, with rectal,
mammary and skin cancer, but not on a wide scale.   More
thought needs to be given to the provision of training and
facilities for surgeons wishing to work predominantly in the
cancer field, as many now intend to do.

The comprehensive cancer specialist, who deals with all
aspects of diagnosis and management of the disease, cannot
be envisaged.   The subject is too broad for that.   There
is no reason, however, why the three natural categories of
specialists should not co-exist and work closely together as
a group.

The radiotherapists recently have changed the title of
their departments to "Radiotherapy and Oncology."   This is
a pity and is misleading.   Radiotherapy is part of oncology
and oncology is not exclusively the province of the
radiotherapist.   The term, Radiological Oncology, would
have been more appropriate and in keeping with modern
requirements.   Such departments of radiological oncology
would be staffed by persons primarily concerned with
radiation therapy of all varieties, which must continue to
have a growing and vital role in treating cancer, and, where
appropriate, with local and systemic chemotherapy of the
disease.

Medical oncology will attract to its ranks physicians
who have a special interest and training in cancer.   As the
place of drug therapy in all forms of malignant disease
becomes clearer, their role will grow in stature.   It is a
great credit to the Royal College of Physicians that the need
for specialist medical oncologists has been recognised so
readily and that the beginning of training programmes are
emerging for interested physicians.

Despite the emergence of a specialist Association of
Surgical Oncology, surgeons have fallen somewhat behind in
their planning.   The needs as far as surgeons are concerned
are clear.   A few selected academic posts are required for
those wishing to specialise whole-time in the subject within
a university department.   Adequate provision must also be
made for oncological instruction for all general surgeons
who are likely to be required to treat patients with cancer

in their daily work.

Perhaps the most important requirement, however, concerns those surgeons who intend to make oncology a predominant part of their practice, be they designated general surgeons, urologists or gynaecologists. Some, in fact, pursue this aim to a point where their practices become almost entirely oncological. Evidence that the demand for this type of specialisation is growing is seen in the enthusiastic younger membership of the recently formed British Association of Surgical Oncology.

To meet this demand, one major step needs to be taken, initiated by the Department of Health and recognised and supported by the Royal College of Surgeons. This step is the provision in the major hospitals around the country for the appointment of at least one consultant surgeon with a declared predominant interest in oncology. The particular regional interest of the person concerned would not matter, be it head and neck, abdominal, urological or some other. Nor would the individual expect, or be expected, to deal with all the surgical cancer work in the hospital. The important thing is that he would be the recognised surgical oncologist in the hospital, and, as such, would relate closely to the other oncologists in the hospitals and through his cancer practice would act as a focal point for educational and administrative oncological activities within the institute.

The distribution of surgical oncologists throughout the country would create a situation around which clinical cancer research and training would flourish, on a national scale. It would also encourage community educational activities in a way which has not been possible hitherto. I believe this development, therefore, to be more imperative than the establishment of other major oncological centres or designated cancer hospitals, however desirable these may be in the long term.

All effort in the cancer field, be it public or professional education, clinical or laboratory research, or the advancement of all aspects of patient care, must revolve around good clinical practice. Malignant diseases, regrettably, are still very common. Without wishing to sound parochial, I must emphasise that the great majority of patients still come under the care of surgeons. There is no

reason to suppose that this situation will change in the
foreseeable future.   Indeed, with increasing emphasis on
earlier diagnosis of all forms of cancer, the role of
surgery is likely to increase rather than decrease.

The response of surgeons to this responsibility and to
the massive challenge of modern oncology has not been
sufficiently vigorous.   Without a determined effort by the
surgical fraternity to participate in the cancer problem,
generously supported by the Department of Health and Social
Security, attempts to re-organise cancer work in a meaningful
way will not succeed.   Where the responsibility lies is
clear, namely, fairly and squarely with the surgeons.
Should they decline this challenge, all hope of improving
the lot of the patient with cancer will vanish.

DISCUSSION

Question 1.   This question is from a lady of the
Women's Cancer Control Campaign.   My association is
primarily concerned with the education of women to seek
early diagnosis of cervical and breast cancer - and yet an
"enlightened" colleague - a school nurse - died recently of
cervical cancer although she had had a "negative" smear test
six months previously.   Is there any way of preventing this
type of tragedy?   I realise that it is difficult, without
knowing the case history, to deal with this specifically but
we would welcome any assurance that can be given that our
efforts to encourage women to seek early diagnosis, are
really worthwhile.

Answer.   This relates somewhat to the point made by
Mr. Baum of the very small tumour in the breast and
widespread metastatic disease with early death.   In the
case of the patient referred to by the questioner, it may be
that the original report was incorrect, but more likely that
the patient had one of these fulminating types of cancer.
Fortunately, such cases are very uncommon and their occurrence
should not detract from the undoubted value of screening in
general.

Question 2.   Are there adequate training schemes in
operation in the United Kingdom for training in oncology?

Answer.   Presumably you mean professional and the answer is, No, except for trainee radiotherapists.

Mr. Raven: How do you propose to develop them?

Well, I think this must be done without any question through the various Royal Colleges.   There are no other organisations who are authoritative enough to put this into practice.   I indicated in my paper that the physicians have begun to take action, but the surgeons have yet so to do. It would be presumptuous of me to talk about the radiotherapists, who already have a very effective administrative organisation.   From the surgeon's point of view, if we are to encourage a generation of young surgeons with a predominant interest in cancer, who would be able to handle the administrative problems of cancer as well as the clinical ones, then there has got to be some form of defined specialist training, and this has yet to be established.

ENCOURAGEMENT FROM RECENT STATISTICS

A.M. Adelstein

Chief Medical Statistician,
Office of Population Censuses and Surveys

INTRODUCTION

In England and Wales most of the central national
records, which together form the health information system,
are managed by the Office of Population Censuses and Surveys
(OPCS).   Two other important systems of records (The Mental
Health Enquiry and Sick Absence Records) are managed by the
Department of Health and Social Security (DHSS).

The Medical Division of OPCS is an integral part of the
Office and much of its work depends on the system of records,
which OPCS manages as part of its general responsibilities
(e.g. the registration of vital events).   The Division is
concerned with the organisation and analysis of data useful
for studying the health (and health problems) of the
community, for research and for administration.   Our work
takes two main forms: first, production and interpretation
of the statistics themselves;   and, second, studies of
particular topics by use of records that have been suitably
organised and indexed.

CURRENT STATISTICAL SYSTEMS

The earliest statistical sources were the census and
registrations of births, deaths and marriages.   Over the
years records from medical services have been added: the
Cancer Registry and the Hospital In-patient Enquiry,
Notification of Infective Diseases and, more recently, of
Congenital Malformations.   The merger of the GRO with the

Government Social Survey in 1970 added the information
collected in the General Household Survey and many specific
surveys.   Furthermore, in 1970 we also began a study of
consultations in general practice.   Finally, a system of
records, which has significance for cancer records and for
cohort studies, is the National Health Service Central
Register (NHSCR) which is basically a clearing house for
registration of the patients of general practitioners in the
National Health Service.

Many of these sources are derived from records created
primarily for various services or for administrative or legal
purposes, not for statistics.   These general information
systems based on services (including registrations of births
and deaths) are the backbone of the national health information
system;   they are valuable in their own right but the
potential of these records can only be achieved by exploiting
them fully - (a) as general descriptive statistics in
themselves;   (b) as general longitudinal statistics by
linking records of persons within and among record systems;
(c) by using the records in retrospective and prospective
studies for problem-orientated research;   and, (d) by ad hoc
research co-ordinated with the basic routine statistics.

CANCER RECORDS

Information on cancer is available from most of the
sets of records listed above, and its potential use is
greatly improved if the records of individual persons are
linked.   The oldest and most reliable records are from
certification of causes of death.   Records of the Hospital
In-patient Enquiry, of General Practice, and from the General
Household Survey all include information on cancer.

CANCER REGISTRATION

This service began as a separate nationwide enterprise
in 1939 and its facilities would be made available for
diagnosis and treatment of cancer.   The register was
transferred to the General Register Office in 1948.

RECENT TRENDS

Since my subject is the encouragement to be found from recent statistics, I shall examine some of the trends in mortality and survival from cancer; some, but not all, of these trends are encouraging - perhaps the most encouraging being the statistical evidence, from this country and others, that cancer is related to life style and environment; that the incidence of every type of cancer varies greatly between countries; that within countries it varies between classes, such as, those based on socio-economic or occupational criteria; that for virtually every type of cancer it is possible to find a place where it is rare; and that there are many examples of its decline.

I shall examine the statistics of deaths attributed to cancer.   Reliable records of causes of death have been available for much longer than have records of live persons with cancer, which can be used to assess the expectation of life (as survival) of cancer cases.   Figure 1 shows how the death rates from cancer of various sites have changed since 1954.   Because the proportions of persons in the different age groups change over time, the rates have been age-standardised, and the results are given as indices with a base of 100 in 1954.

Fig. 1 shows that the trends of mortality have been downward for four major sites of cancer and upward for six: rates have been declining for cancer of the stomach, colon and rectum, mouth and pharynx, and for cancer of the cervix uteri in women; but they have been increasing from cancer of the lung and bronchus, pancreas, breast, ovary, prostate, and from leukaemia.   Mortality from cancer of the oesophagus of men declined until 1963 and then increased, while in women it has been increasing slowly.

Because the standardised figure measures the rate for all persons taken together, it may, sometimes, conceal differing trends between age groups.   This happens, for example, in mortality from cancer of the lung and bronchus, as explained later.   Furthermore, since cancer, like some other chronic diseases, may appear many years after the initial stimulus - as much as 40 years after exposure to some asbestos dusts - the interpretation of mortality trends over time needs to take account of variations between ages,

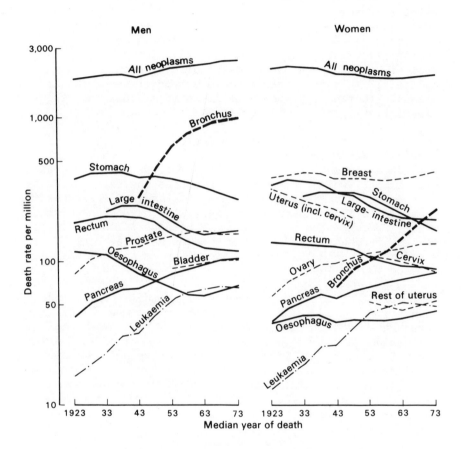

Fig. 1

between periods, and between generations (sometimes called
cohorts).   A cohort in this context refers to a group of
persons born in a defined period, say a decade.   If death
rates change over time, it may be possible to separate the
effects of age, period, and cohort, and thus to correlate
the changing rates with environmental factors which may have
stamped their mark (bad or good) on the members of a
generation many years before the effect is seen in (changed)
mortality.   The fact that mortality rates (and incidence) of
many specific cancers rise with age, within cohorts, is
itself an indication that environmental factors (carcinogens)
may be responsible, their effect being related to how much
and for how long persons were exposed.   Epidemiologists have
spoken of a "cohort effect" when the pattern of mortality
between ages is similar in each generation, and the general
level of mortality in each cohort reflects the result of
early influences.

COHORT ANALYSIS

The Registrar General has recently published a new and
up-to-date version of Case's original tables showing death
rates in England and Wales for 36 primary cancers from 1911
to 1970 in 5-year age groups in successive 5-year periods,
each table extending as far back as the classification of
disease permits. (1)

I shall now analyse mortality statistics for England and
Wales from 1911 to 1970 of one of the primary cancers,
bronchus and lung, shown in the quinary - quinquiennial form
in graphs.

The horizontal axis of Figure 2 shows the central
position of the range of dates of birth of successive cohorts
(not, as is usual, showing dates of death) in order to make
the inter-relationship between age, period and cohort clearer.
The death rates for cohorts are shown on the vertical axis on
a log scale;   thus for the cohort born around 1906 the rates
at successive ages are on the vertical path upwards from the
1906 point on the abscissa.   (The last point is the average
for 4 years, 1971-1974).

Consider the graph showing mortality of men: the
general impression is of more or less parallel lines rising

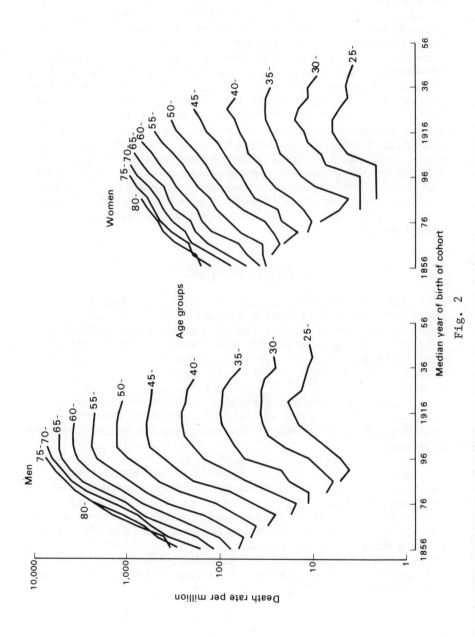

Fig. 2

steadily in each age group of the generations born up to about 1900; for later cohorts (recall that the rates are on a log scale) the curves reach a plateau, and then the most recent points for age groups under 65-69 turn down, the curves maintaining their more or less parallel arrangement; of course, for each successively younger age group the curve ends at one stop to the right, since the next cohort has not yet reached the later age.   The distinct turn down in the age group (40-44) begins in the cohort born around 1920. For earlier cohorts (born before 1906) now over 65, the rates for females continue upwards to their end.

Mortality rates of women from cancer of lung and bronchus are shown in Figure 2.   Some of the trends are similar to those of the men, but there are also considerable differences. Above the age of 45 the trend over the whole period has been consistently upward, but at a lower level than for men. (For example, at age 50-54 the rate for men is more than 7 times higher.)   For younger women, below 35, the graphs resemble those of men, but at a lower level.   The peak mortality for women under 35 was in the cohorts born about 1921-1926, after which there is a turn down (for men it was in the 1916 cohort.)   This turn down began about 1950 but had become clear after 1955.   Note that the decline from the peak is related to age; the younger the greater the relative decline, and it is very much less than the rise which preceded it in successive generations up to those who were born around 1926.

Even though a great deal of the rise of mortality rates shown in the census must have been the result of improved diagnosis, the pattern (or mortality) is consistent with a cohort effect, which is interrupted by a smaller period effect.   The cohort picture is shown by the parallel lines, first the rise, then the plateau, and finally a decline in the younger age group.   The period effect is shown by the slight loss of the regular parallelism so that the peaks in the age groups change for successive cohorts.   The curves of male mortality in the age group 55-59 reach a peak in 1901 cohort; the 45-49 age group in the 1911 cohort; the 30-34 year-olds in the 1916 cohort.   This moving peak suggests a period effect which produced a reduction of mortality about the late 1950's.   The figures of female mortality also show a cohort pattern.   These cohort trends would be consistent with the effect of an increasing exposure of a carcinogen begun early and continued throughout life.

This is an old story, and everyone here will be familiar
with the idea that cigarette smoking is the main cause.
The idea is, of course, based on much more than juxtaposing
these figures to those of cigarette consumption.   There is
an extensive network of evidence to substantiate the
relationship between smoking and lung cancer. (2)

But what about the recent decline in rates?   To try to
answer this I will examine the two environmental factors,
smoking and air pollution.

CIGARETTES CONSUMED BY SUCCESSIVE GENERATIONS

Todd has analysed the smoking patterns by cohorts of
men and women adjusting the data to take account of tar
content and filters. (3)   Fig. 3, taken from Todd's analysis
shows the lifetime consumption of cigarettes by cohorts of
men and women.   Although the information available was
somewhat sketchy when surveys were first begun (taking these
figures at face value) it appears that the total number of
cigarettes consumed over the life of the average individual
of the successive cohorts reached a peak (in most age groups)
in the cohorts of men born around 1915 and 1920.   The 1930
cohort has a distinctly lower average consumption than
previous cohorts and this decline seems to have continued in
later cohorts.   But the decline is small compared to the
previous rise, and the main impression is of a prolonged
plateau followed by a small decline.   The trend to increasing
smoking by women began later than that of men and was
interrupted by a plateau in the cohorts born around 1925,
1930 and 1935, and, though the increase continues, consumption
by women is still lower than by men.

AIR POLLUTION

The role of an urban factor (not necessarily air
pollution) in lung cancer was reviewed in a report by the
Royal College of Physicians.   After allowing for different
smoking practices, differences in mortality between urban and
rural areas,between countries, and between immigrants and
home populations, suggest that air pollution has an effect
though it is much smaller than that of cigarettes.   Air
pollution by smoke from domestic use of coal declines

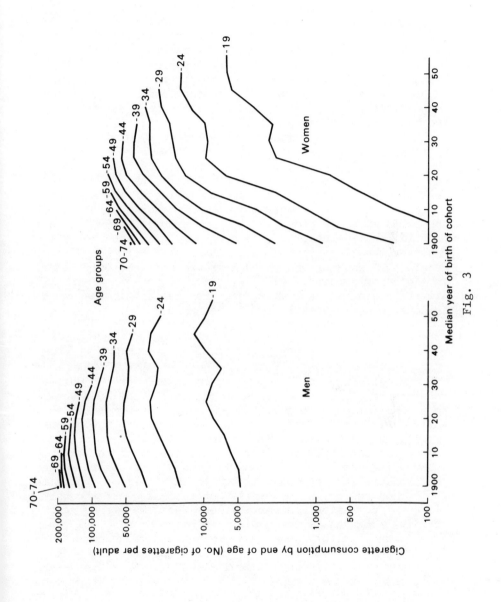

Fig. 3

gradually after reaching a peak during the First World War, and the decline accelerated after the introduction of the clean air act of the mid-1950's. (5)   Thus two causes of lung cancer, smoking and air pollution, reinforce one another; but at any particular time the relative impact of each varied between the sexes.   For men the peak of smoking and the peak of air pollution were experienced by roughly the same cohorts; generations born after 1920 were beginning to breathe less pollution and to smoke less.   Of course, there is no exact point at which the changing effect of the two hazards on the generations is clear cut; generations born at progressively longer times before 1920 will have spent proportionately more of their lives in polluted air. Thus, succeeding generations are affected by both a period and a cohort effect, and this is reflected by the way the peak of cancer incidence by cohorts varies in the age groups of men.   The peak of mortality is not reached by the same cohort in each age group; older age groups (55-59) reach a peak in the 1901 cohort; the 45-49 age group in the 1911 cohort; the 30-34 year-olds in the cohort born in 1916. Recall that smoking in some age groups declined only later, in the cohorts born after 1925.   The reduction of mortality, after its peak in each age group, is greatest in the young persons, reaching nearly 50% in men aged 25-29.

MORTALITY OF MEN

The effect of diminishing air pollution on successive generations of men after those born, say, about 1900 would be a combination of a cohort and a period effect.   In the early part of this century successive generations would be exposed in their early lives to increasing pollution; but the decreasing exposure after 1920 would affect the older ages of the same cohorts; and the age of the cohort at which the exposure was less than it was in the previous generation would then reduce in successive generations.   If the harmful effect of pollution was more or less the same at any age, then the lung cancer rate (all else being equal) would turn down at successively lower ages in successive cohorts.   That this happens to some degree is shown by the way the peak mortality moves from generation to generation.   The steady improvement of the atmosphere after 1920 was accelerated by the Clean Air Act.   The effect of either of these would show as a period change on the cohort curves.   On the other hand, the effect of cigarette smoking, the main cause, reached a peak for the cohorts of men born about 1920-1925, and declined somewhat thereafter.

Cohorts of men born after 1920 have experienced progressively less of both air pollution and cigarette tar; as for the earlier generations this shows in the death rates as a combination of cohort and period effect. Here, as for the older men, the peak rate shifts to the right in younger ages; in the 35-39 year-old men the peak is in the 1916 cohort, while in the 25-29's it is in the 1921 cohort; and in the 20-24's in the 1926 cohort.

On this hypothesis the observed changes in lung cancer mortality for men are compatible with the combination of the known changes in air pollution and cigarette smoking. The decline of mortality is as yet small compared with the preceding rise. In middle-aged men, it could be entirely the result of diminished pollution. In younger men, there could be the added effect of less cigarette tar. The younger the men the more marked is the relative decline, which is what we might expect because they would have spent more of their lives in relatively clean air.

MORTALITY OF WOMEN

The steep rise in cigarette smoking by women took place in successive cohorts born after the turn of the century; the steep increase by men was in cohorts born before 1900.

The turn round of formerly rising mortality rates is confined to women under 44 years of age, the age reached by the 1931 cohort in 1970-74, the last point on the graphs; female mortality has benefitted from a lull in the rising trend of smoking in the 3 cohorts of 1925, 1930 and 1935; these and later cohorts born about 1940 could have benefitted from relatively increasingly clean air - children born after 1960 or thereabouts could have a whole life free of serious air pollution; the older a person was in 1960, the more he would already have been exposed.

The downturn in rates of mortality of women began in the young ages, under 30, and has now reached the 40-45 year age group whereas that of men reaches even the 65-69 year-old

group.   The decline in both sexes is greatest in the young
persons, though small compared with the previous rise.
Progressively cleaner air may have more effect on young
persons if only because it would influence a greater
proportion of their lives.   That air pollution has been a
major factor in both the rise and now the decline of
mortality of both sexes can hardly be doubted - but its
effect is considerably less than that of smoking.   The
reduction of mortality to about one half its highest peak
seems possible.   It is not clear how much of the most recent
fall in mortality is the result of the reduction in tobacco
tar because there has not yet been enough time for the effect
to emerge clearly.   Also, the correction which takes account
of tar content was applied only to figures after 1965, whereas
the change to filtered cigarettes began somewhat earlier.
For this discussion I have taken the figures published by Todd
at face value.

    In summary, for both men and women the mortality from
lung cancer over time could be related to the combined effect
of smoking and air pollution - the former having the dominant
role, - when age, generation and period are taken into account.
Successive cohorts of men increased their smoking before women
did, and during the period when air pollution was rising, so
that they suffered increasingly from the effects of both.
By the time air pollution began to diminish, smoking in men
had reached near to its highest point;   soon after this the
effect of increasing clean air was apparent.   Women, however,
experienced their major rise in smoking later and after the
air pollution had begun to decline so that their rates of
lung cancer continued to rise after that of men was declining.
But the rates of mortality of women are still much lower age
for age.

    Two other analyses of the national mortality figures
gives clues to the effects of environment and life styles on
lung cancer;   the first is by geographic area and the second,
which extends over many years, is by socio-economic classes
based on occupation.

URBANISATION

    Figures 4 and 5 show, in cohort form, the mortality from
lung cancer in 5 categories of urbanisation.   As is well-
known there is a regular gradient with urbanisation.

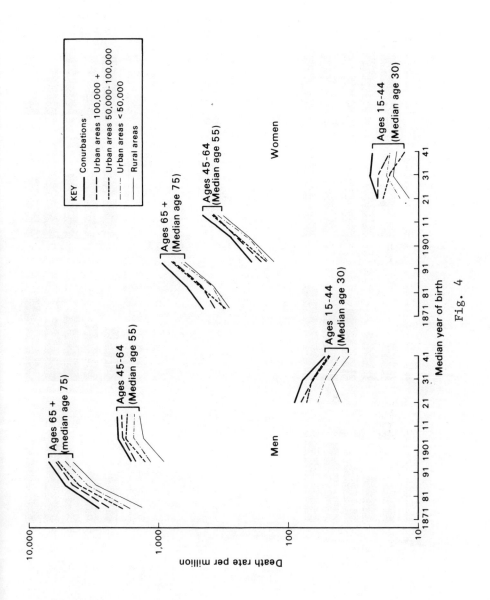

Fig. 4

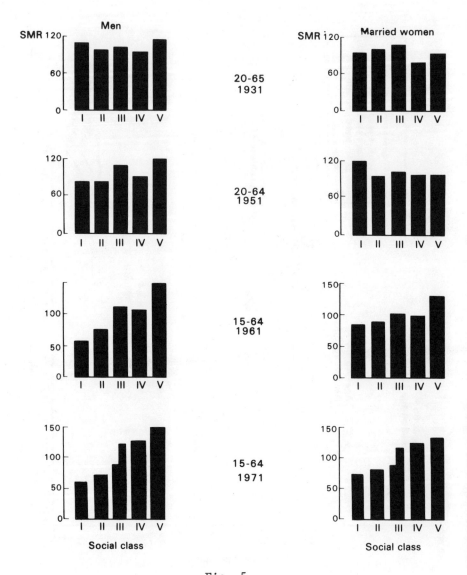

Fig. 5

Reduction in mortality of males occurred first in the
smaller towns, and last in the rural areas.   Their wives'
mortality diminished later (as discussed earlier) and the
first to be affected were women in middle-sized towns.
Interpreting these figures is not straightforward because
there is not sufficient information on differences of
smoking, and on the effectiveness of clean air acts between
town and country.   Some authorities have suggested that the
later and smaller effect in rural areas is the result of
there being less change in pollution during this period.

SOCIO-ECONOMIC DIFFERENCES IN MORTALITY

Figure 5[*] shows mortality rates from cancer of the lung
(SMRS) at census periods in the five categories of social
class described by the Registrar General. (6)   The analyses
based on the 1951 census is known to have an error which
increased the death rate of social class I at the expense of
II by wrongly classifying company directors.   Nevertheless,
the overall picture is clear.   In the early results (1931)
the differences in mortality from cancer of the lung and
bronchus between the classes were small and irregular.
Around 1951 gradients appeared between the classes from I to
V, viz., up for men and down for women. Around 1961 and
again around 1971 the gradient of mortality between the
classes (I-V) increases noticeably for men; having reached
the range of SMRs from 42 to 144 for women the gradient
downward from I to V in 1951 changed in 1961 to an upward
one, as it was for men, and by 1971 it had widened
considerably.   Interpretation of time trends of mortality
between social classes is bedevilled by changes in the
composition of the classes;   changes which are the result of
altered lists of occupations which constitute the classes,
as well as changes in the numbers of persons in the various
occupations.   For example, as social class V (unskilled)
becomes smaller over time, its mortality is more influenced
by groups who, as it were, cannot get out because of poor
health.   The increase of the range of SMRs (all causes)
between classes, which took place around 1961 and has
persisted, could be, at least partly, a result of the transfer
of relatively healthy persons into class IV from V.   As the
figure shows, there was no gradient between SMRs of classes
in 1931.   However, SMRs may mask differences in particular

* Figures of mortality by social class based on 1971 census
  are provisional.

age groups; and at that time (1931) the male mortality from
lung cancer below the age of 44 was already highest in social
class V and by 1951 it appeared to be so below 64.

While the mortality rate (from lung cancer) for all men
below 45 declined between the studies based on the censuses
of 1951 and 1961, the decline in class I was steeper, and
for men aged 45-54 the decline was noted only in social class
I.*   Interpreting the changes over time in the mortality
gradient between social classes in relation to smoking is not
straightforward because for figures of cigarette consumption
we rely on small quota samples used in the early surveys of
the TRC.   At their face value, the change to the present
pattern of mortality preceded the change in smoking, which
until about 1960 showed approximately similar numbers of
cigarettes smoked in the various social classes.   But it is
likely that those survey figures underestimate the effective
difference between the classes; they do not take account of
the age at which smoking began, of the length of cigarette
smoked, or of the filters; each of these is likely to have
a social gradient.   Also, the interpretation of the effects
of smoking and of pollution is likely to have a social
gradient.   There is no doubt about the gradient of smoking
between classes after about 1960, since which time a number
of substantial surveys point in the same direction in the UK
and in the USA.   Cigarette consumption is higher and begins
at younger ages consistently from class I to V.

In summary, this analysis of the statistics of cancer
of the lung and bronchus emphasises the point that the age-
standardised rate does not tell the whole story: it is
necessary to examine age specific rates and to take account
of cohorts.   Other cancers for which this applies are
leukaemia of adults and cancer of the cervix uteri. (7, 8)

Analysis of mortality from cancer of the cervix uteri
reveals that within the general downward trend during the
century there are some cohorts of women whose rates are
significantly higher than the corresponding rates of cohorts
before and after.   The cohorts with high rates were women
who were young adults during the war periods, a finding that
is consistent with the known differences in promiscuity.
Mortality from leukaemia in adults rises steeply with age,
and the age-standardised rate over time showing a more or
less stable rate overlooks the declining rates in younger
adults.

CANCER REGISTRY: SURVIVAL RATES

Until 1971 cancer registration at the national level depended on the regional registries for information on both incidence and deaths.   Since then we have been developing a system whereby deaths of registered cases are identified systematically in O.P.C.S. records.   This will enable us to produce regular tables of expectation of life (survival rates) for cancer cases.   In addition, the system will enable us to carry out prospective studies in order to test hypotheses of causes of cancer.

Because the older system of data collection was inevitably slow and improvements in survival have taken place recently, I shall show only survival rates for children's cancer, which have been analysed by quicker methods.   Figures calculated from national records by the Childhood Cancer Research Group of the University of Oxford show the great improvement achieved in the treatment of two particular tumours: 5-year survival from Hodgkin's disease increased from 36 per cent in 1962 to 61 per cent in 1968;   for Wilm's tumour, the corresponding figures are 18 to 35 per cent.

In 1971 the MRC Committee on Leukaemia published figures from national records (with a small deficit) showing the improvement in survival from acute lymphocytic leukaemia among a specially treated group.   Recent (unpublished) figures show that the 3-year survival has reached over 60 per cent in a sample comprising most cases in the country.

SUMMARY

Various national records provide information on cancer, e.g., Cancer Registration, Death Certification, Hospital Records.   From these it is possible to calculate age-standardised mortality rates.   These rates have decreasing trends for five major sites of cancers (stomach, colon and rectum, mouth, cervix uteri and ovary) and increasing trends for four (lung and bronchus, pancreas, prostate and oesophagus.) Age-specific cohort rates reveal contrary trends between ages, between cohorts and between periods.   The rising trend for lung cancer in men has turned down in persons under 60 beginning in the cohorts born after 1920.   For women the turn-down is later and confined to younger persons.   These trends are compatible with the explanation that the main

cause is cigarette smoking supplemented by the effects of
air pollution.   In the case of women the effect of the
general decline in air pollution was swamped by the effect
of cigarette smoking which was then increasing steeply and
continued so until after the second war though at a lower
general level than men.   The evidence shows that cigarette
smoking is the dominant factor, and this is why the rates
of mortality declined earlier for men than for women.
Recently-born cohorts of either sex have rates of lung cancer
mortality that are lower than their peaks by around 30%.
Lung cancer also has an urban/rural gradient; the down-turn
began in the medium-sized towns and was least and last in the
rural areas where there may have been less air pollution.

        The differences in mortality, from lung cancer, between
social classes has changed in both men and women; there is
now a sharp gradient up from I to V.   Figures for earlier
years showed that there was no difference for men, while for
women it was in the reverse direction.

        Five-year percentage survival of children with Hodgkin's
disease, and with Wilm's tumour between 1962 and 1968 have
improved from 36 to 61 and from 18 to 35 respectively.

        I am grateful to the Registrar General for permission
to publish, and to him and other colleagues for their help,
and also to Mr. G. Todd for allowing me to read his paper
before publication.

REFERENCES

1.   Cancer Mortality, England and Wales 1911-1970. Studies
          on Medical and Population Subjects No. 29.
2.   Fletcher, C.M. and Horn, D. 1971. World Health
          Organisation, Smoking and Health.
3.   Todd, G.F. 1975. Changes in Smoking Patterns in the U.K.
          Tobacco Research Council. Occasional Paper 1.
          London.
4.   Todd, G.F. In press. Personal communication.
5.   Pollution and Health. Committee of the Royal College of
          Physicians. London. 1970. Pitman.
6.   The Registrar General's Decennial Supplements, England
          and Wales. Occupational Mortality. H.M.S.O. London.
7.   Hill, G.B. and Adelstein, A.M. 1967. Lancet, p.605.

8.   Adelstein, A.M. and White, G. 1975. Population Trends,
        3. H.M.S.O.
9.   Duration of Survival of Children with Acute Leukaemia.
        British Medical Journal. 1971. 4:7.
10. The General Household Survey. 1972. H.M.S.O.
11. Statistics of Smoking in the United Kingdom. 1969.
        Tobacco Research Council, London.

DISCUSSION

Question 1.   Would Dr. Adelstein agree that important
data about human cancer are being lost to-day because of
imperfect records?   How can this be remedied?

Answer.   I hope that talking about imperfect records
does not suggest that there could be perfect records,
because this would be dreaming.   Nearly all our records on
cancer, as on other diseases, come from medical services;
i.e., they are by-products of notes kept for medical care.
They are NOT designed primarily for statistics and this
paradoxically may be the reason why they are robust.   Our
system of records of cancers for the whole country is, I
believe, a good one, and it is improving.   Soon it will
allow fairly fast monitoring of incidence and of survival;
and it will enable epidemiologists to carry out prospective,
as well as retrospective, studies.   Any local registry is
able to specialise in a direction of its choosing.   So, for
example, South Thames Region analyses more characteristics
than do other regions or the National Registry;   in Manchester
the Childhood Cancer Registry has concentrated on histology,
while the Oxford Childhood Cancer Registry is concerned in
general with children's cancer.   Of course, all our records
need to be examined for quality and system design, but I do
not favour damaging criticism that would result in failure to
use good records while we wait for 'perfect' ones.   It is
important to realise that the limitations and the strength of
this general system should be nurtured so that relevant
hypotheses can be answered, if not by the main system as such,
then by one of the numerous second level systems which it
facilitates.

Question 2.   Could Dr. Adelstein indicate the possible
value of lifelong individual health records commencing at
birth?

Answer.   I would need a long time to answer this
question.   My illustrious predecessor, William Farr, talked
about it in the last century, and we talk a bit about it now:
what we mean, of course, are not detailed records.   It would
be impossible to keep detailed records of people from birth
to death; but we could keep records of important landmarks
in people's lives, and a few institutions are doing that.
We would have liked to do it for all England and Wales, that
is, to put together the records of births, hospital admissions
and deaths, and possibly marriages.   We would like to have
done that but there are two problems and they are the same
two problems which I mentioned before.   One is cost and the
other is confidentiality.   The latter worries some people
to such a degree that we do not think we would be able to do
it.   I nearly said get away with it.   I do not think we
would like to get away with anything.   I think we would
acknowledge that it is absolutely essential to monitor, if
you like to use that word, certain events; for example,
hazards in the environment, in food or some therapies, and
also we need to measure the outcome of various forms of
medical care, and to study the relationship of diseases to
one another and to environment.   When we fail to prevent an
event like the thalidomide disaster, we are asked why.   If,
during a period in which there is no unusual or alarming
event, we say we would like to construct linked records so
that we do not miss worrying signs, we are told, No, because
the records are confidential.   So, the public really has to
make up its own mind about this.   On the one hand there is
the threat to individual privacy; on the other hand the
threat to his health and to that of other people.   We would
like to threaten his privacy a little.   As far as we know,
nobody has suffered from the kind of records we keep and
there has never been to our knowledge anybody that has been
embarrassed by the fact that, potentially, we might know
that certain people have certain diseases.   It is obvious
that, as a basic data set which also enables further research,
we would like to have a system of linked data.   This would
be the greatest advance in medical records.

Question 3.   15 year survival rates are of enormous
importance.   Would Dr. Adelstein agree that they really
mean cure for most cases?

Answer.   I do not think that there is time to tackle
this question in depth.   In practice, for most cancers,
persons who survive, say ten years, have a life expectancy

thereafter similar to the population at large (taking account of age); this can be interpreted as cure for the survivors, on average.   A notable exception is cancer of the breast; the mortality rates on average continue at a higher level than the equivalent population.   On the other hand, if these calculations were carried out on data from patients with early stages of breast cancer, they would show that they would survive much longer.

DELEGATE LIST, SYMPOSIA 1975 & 1976

Name	Title	Qualifications	Affiliation
Abbott	Miss M.	SRN, SCM, HV, RMN	South Glamorgan AHA
Abranovitz	Rev. C.		Leeds AHA
Adams	Miss J.	DSRT	Leicester Royal Infirmary
Adams	Mrs. K.M.	MCSP	St. Luke's Hospital, Guildford
Adams	Mrs. R.	SRN, RCNT, DN	Middlesex Hospital, London
Ager	Mrs. D.M.	SRN, RCNT	North Surrey AHA
Alden	Mrs. G.M.		Barking and Havering AHA
Alexander	K.		Research Department, MCMF
Allen	B.A.	SRN, RMN, DN	Bedfordshire AHA
Al-Sanjari	Mrs. E.D.	SRN, SCM, HV	Mount Vernon Hospital, Middlesex
Alsworth	Mrs. M.L.	SRN	Greenwich and Bexley AHA
Amherst	* Lord	CBE	Honorary Treasurer, MCMF
Anderson	* Dr. D.J.	MB, Ch.B, FFCM, DPH	Welsh Office
Anderson	Mrs. J.R.	Nursing Officer	North Hertfordshire HD
Angeli	Mrs. N.	Nursing Officer	St. Peter's Hospital, Chertsey
Anglesio	Dr. E.		Torino, Italy
Angwin	Miss J.B.	SRN, SCM, QN, HV	Clwyd AHA
Aranguren	Dr. G.		University Hospital, Caracas
Archer	Mrs. J.	SRN, RMN, CMP(Pt I)	Grove Park Hospital, London
Armstrong	Miss M.	MA(Cantab), SRN	St. Bartholomew's Hospital, London
Arnold	Miss H.W.	SRN, SCM, QN, HV	Hampshire AHA
Ashe	B.	SRN, RMN, RNT	Harlow School of Nursing, Essex
Askham	Mrs. I.G.		Executive, MCMF
Atkinson	Miss R.	SRN, SCM, HV	St. Thomas's HD
Attwood	Mrs. I.E.	Social Worker	Age Concern
Attwood	Miss L.M.	Medical Secretary	London
Austin	Miss G.M.	SRN, SCM, ONC	St. Mary's Hospital, London
Axe	Miss J.M.	SRN, CMB(Pt I), HV	Linton Hospital, Maidstone

Bailey	Mrs. I	Social Worker	Kettering General Hospital, Northants
Bailey	Mrs. I	SRN	Manfield Hospital, Northampton
Baird	Miss V.A.	SRN	St. Mary's Hospital, London
Baker	G.	HND	Research Department, MCMF
Baker	Miss M.	SRN	Hammersmith Hospital, London
Baker	Mrs. M.	Social Worker	Frimley Park Hospital, Surrey
Baker	Miss R.A.B.	RSCN, SRN, MTD, HV, QN	Executive Committee, MCMF
Baldeo	G.	SRN	St. James's Hospital, London
Banks	H.D.	SRN, StD	School of Nursing, Hastings
Barlow	Miss J.M.	SRN, DSR(T)	Middlesex Hospital, London
Barnes	Mrs. C.	SRN, SCM, RCNT	Dorset AHA
Barnes	Miss D.M.	SRN, SCM, RCNT	Royal Infirmary, Bristol
Barnes	Mrs. D.M.	SRN, SCM, HV	Buckinghamshire AHA
Barnes	Miss M.	SRN	Royal Marsden Hospital, Surrey
Barnett	Mrs. M.P.		Research Department, MCMF
Barrett	Mrs. M.A.	SRN	West Sussex AHA
Basu	Dr. T.K.	BSc, BVSc, MSc, PhD	Research Department, MCMF
Bates	Miss M.	SRN, RSCN	St. Bartholomew's Hospital, London
Bates	Mrs. S.	CQSW	General Hospital, Oldham
Beardmore	Miss I	SRN, RSCN, ONC, RNT	Sunderland AHA
Beatson	* Dr. J.H.	MB, ChB	Westbury-on-Trym, Bristol
Beaumont	Miss J.	Nursing Officer	Hertfordshire AHA
Bebbington	Mrs. J.K.		National Society for Cancer Relief
Bee	Miss E.J.	SRN	St. Bartholomew's Hospital, London
Beechey	Mrs. M.P.	MSRT	Churchill Hospital, Oxford
Bell	Mrs. B.	SRN, SCM	Buckinghamshire AHA
Bell	G.	MB, ChB, FRCSG, ChM	Royal Infirmary, Greenock
Bennett	Dr. M.B.	MRCS, LRCP, DMR(Lond)	Groote Schuur Hospital, South Africa
Bennette	Dr. G.	MA, MB, BChir	British Cancer Council
Bentley	Dr. G.C.	MB, ChB, DRCOG	Derbyshire Family Practitioner Committee

Bentley		Mrs. N.M.	RGN, SCM, HV	Manchester AHA(T)
Berman	*	Miss A.	SRN, RCNT, Dip.N	Middlesex Hospital, London
Berry		Miss E.M.	SRN, SCM	Essex AHA
Best		Miss J.	SRN, SCM, HV	Radiotherapy Hospital, Cookridge
Bevan		Mrs. J.	SRN, NCDN	Gwent AHA
Bevan		J.E.	SRN, DN	Greenwich and Bexley AHA
Beynon		Mrs. I.M.	Nursing Officer	Dyfed AHA
Bhatt		Mrs. K.K.	BA, Cert.App.Soc.Stud.	General Hospital, Newcastle-upon-Tyne
Biddulph		Miss C.	Nursing Officer	Manchester AHA(T)
Billimoria		Dr. B.M.	MB, BS, DRCOG	Kingston and Richmond AHA
Birchall		Mrs. J.	SRN, HV	Nottinghamshire AHA(T)
Bird		J.F.	SRN	Essex AHA
Bishun	*	Dr. N.P.	BSc, PhD, FRSH	Research Department, MCMF
Blackburn		Mrs. G.M.	SRN	Ipswich Hospital, Suffolk
Blackett		S/Ldr. J.B.	AFC	Cancer Research Campaign, London
Blakebrough		Mrs. K.	Nursing Officer	Barking and Havering AHA
Blakey		Mrs. E.I.	Clinical Teacher	Hertfordshire AHA
Blakey		Miss M.J.	BA, CQSW	Royal Infirmary, Bristol
Blayney		Miss M.	Social Worker	St. Thomas's Hospital, London
Bollas		Mrs. S.	MSW	Royal National Orthopaedic Hospital, London
Borg	*	Miss M.A.	SRN, SCM, Dip.Soc.	London
Bothwell	*	Miss P.	SRN, RSCN	Edenhall Nursing Home, MCMF
Botley		Miss P.M.	SRN, BTA	Croydon AHA
Boulian		D.	MSW	Hammersmith Hospital, London
Bowley		Miss J.	SRN	Wessex AHA
Bradshaw		Dr. E.M.	MB, ChB, MRCS, LRCP	Syston, Leicestershire
Bradshaw		Dr. J.D.	MB, ChB, FRCP	Royal Infirmary, Leicester
Brain	*	Lady A.		Executive Committee, MCMF
Brandwood		A.	SRN	St. Ann's Hospital, London

Breeze	Mrs. C.D.	SRN	Domiciliary Nursing Service, MCMF
Brewer	Miss R.M.	MSCP	White Lodge Centre, Chertsey
Bridge	Miss B.P.	SRN, SCM, RCT	Philip Templeman School of Nursing, Poole
Bringan	Dr. J.W.	LRCP,LRCS,MFCM,DPH	Northern RHA
Britton	Miss B.	HV	Worcester HD
Broadbent	Dr. A.R.	MFCM, DPH, DIH	Ealing, Hammersmith and Hounslow AHA
Broderick	Miss M.M.	SRN, HV	Royal Marsden Hospital, Surrey
Bromfield	Mrs. W.J.	MSW	St. Alban's City Hospital
Bromley	Mrs. B.	SRN	Abingdon Hospital, Oxfordshire
Brons	Mrs. A.	Social Worker	St. Charles's Hospital, London
Brookes	* Mrs. D.	SRN, SCM	Warren Pearl House, MCMF
Brookes	R.	FRCS, FRCS.Ed.	Royal Infirmary, Chester
Brophy	Miss B.	SRN	St.Joseph's Convalescent Home, Bournemouth
Brown	Miss H.A.	RGN	Lothian Health Board
Brown	Miss H.J.	Social Worker	Harold Wood Hospital, Essex
Brown	Miss J.	SRN, RSCN, SCM	King's College Hospital, London
Brownhill	Miss G.E.	SRN, SCM, HV, QN	Cheltenham HD
Buchanan	Miss M.	RGN, SCM, QN, HV	Humberside AHA
Buck	A.E.	Nursing Officer	Tunbridge Wells HD
Buckland	Miss D.L.		Department of Energy, London
Bullen	Miss J.	RGN, SCM	Ninewells Hospital, Dundee
Bullivant	Mrs. S.A.	SRN, ONC, QN	Merton, Sutton and Wandsworth AHA
Bunting	Miss J.J.	CSW	Kettering Hospital, Northants
Burd	* Mrs. H.F.	MCSP	Women's Cancer Control Campaign
Burdge	Mrs. L.S.	SRN	Royal Marsden Hospital, London
Burns	Miss K.	SRN	South London Hospital
Burr	Miss S.	BA	St. Thomas's Hospital, London
Burrell	Mrs. J.M.	MCSP	Birmingham

Butler	* Mrs. J.	MP	House of Commons, London
Butterworth	Miss B.A.	SRN, RMN, RCNT	Middlesex Hospital, London
Callaway	Mrs. M.	SRN	Wexham Park Hospital, Berkshire
Cameron	Dr. A.D.	MB, MFCM, DPH	Lambeth, Southwark & Lewisham AHA(T)
Cameron	Miss L.	RFN, RGN, SCM	Belvedere Hospital, Glasgow
Camm	* Dr. C.E.	MB,BS,DPH,DIH,MFCM	Oxford RHA
Campbell	Dr. B		East Grinstead, Sussex
Campbell	* Dr. I.D.	MB,ChB,FRCPE,FFCM	Lothian Health Board
Campbell	* Miss J.P.		Homes Sub-Committee, MCMF
Cann	Miss M.E.	SRN	West Birmingham HD
Cannell	Mrs. C.J.	SRN, CMB(PtI)	Royal National Throat, Nose and Ear Hospital, London
Cannon	P.G.	Nursing Officer	Medway HD
Capper	Miss E.	SRN, SCM, DN	St. Bartholomew's Hospital, London
Carey	M.	SRN	General Hospital, Cheltenham
Carman	Mrs. M.F.	SRN, DN	Dartford and Gravesend HD
Carpenter	Mrs. J.M.	SRN, CMB(PtI)	Southend HD
Carpenter	Miss P.R.	SRN, SCM, RNCT	Greenwich and Bexley AHA
Carstairs	Mrs. M.	Social Worker	General Hospital, Kettering
Carter	Miss D.	CQSW	City of Westminster
Carter	Miss L.V.	SRN	Middlesex Hospital, London
Carter	Mrs. M	Nursing Officer	South Tees HD
Cartmell	* Miss H.V.	B.Soc.Sc.,Dip.S.W.	West Birmingham HD
Carver	Miss L.	Assistant Matron	Chest Hospital, Benenden
Case	Dr. E.M.	MA, PhD	British Cancer Council
Cassells	Miss S.M.	SRN, SCM	St. Bartholomew's Hospital, London
Castle	Mrs. E.J.	SRN, HV, FWT	South East Kent HD
Castle	Miss E.J.	SRN	Westminster Hospital, London
Cattell	Mrs. P.A.	HDSRT	Royal Marsden Hospital, London

Chamberlain	Dr. J.	MB, BS, DCH, MFCM	University College Hospital Medical School, London
Chang	S.	HDSRT	Hammersmith Hospital, London
Chapman	Mrs. D.M.	SRN, QN	Dorset AHA
Chapman	* Mrs. V.A.	BA, CQSW	Social Services Department, Coventry
Chaput de Saintonge	Mrs. E.N.	Social Worker	Royal Marsden Hospital, London
Charlton	* Dr. A.	BA, PhD	Manchester Regional Committee for Cancer Education
Chivers	Miss E.	SRN	Queen Mary's Hospital, Sidcup
Clapham	Miss J.	BSc, SRN	Manchester AHA
Clark	Mrs. D.	Dip.Soc.Stud.,CIA	Social Services Department, Wiltshire
Clark	* Dr. J.S.	MB, BS	Conrad House, MCMF
Clark	Miss M.	SRN	Weston Park Hospital, Sheffield
Clarke	Rev. J.P.		Leeds Infirmary
Clarkson	Mrs. B.M.	SRN, NDN Cert.	East Dorset HD
Clayton	Miss R.	SRN, SCM, HV	Ealing,Hammersmith and Hounslow AHA
Cleak	Miss G.	Nursing Officer	Westminster Hospital, London
Clifford	Mrs. L.A.	CQSW	West Middlesex Hospital
Cobby	Miss M.	SRN	Enfield and Harringay AHA
Coffey	Miss R.A.	MSW	North Middlesex Hospital
Cogan	Mrs. H.E.	SRN	Colchester HD
Coleman	Dr. F.B.	MA,BM,BCh,DRCOG	Market Deeping, Lincolnshire
Collins	Miss B.	Nursing Officer	Barking and Havering AHA
Collins	Miss M.	SRN	Whittington Hospital, London
Collins	Miss Z.H.	SRN, RCNT	Nightingale School of Nursing,London
Collyer	Miss P.	SRN,SCM,HV, Dip.Soc.Sc.,FRSH	Health Education Council, London
Columb	Miss M.B.	Clinical Tutor	Hammersmith Hospital, London
Comerford	M.	RFN, DN	Moffat Child Health Centre, London

Compton	Lady	SRN, SCM	Executive Committee, MCMF
Conlon	Sister J.		Ulster Cancer Foundation
Conquest	* Mrs. N.		Research Department, MCMF
Cook	Mrs. D.	MCSP	Chelmsford HD
Cooke	Dr. M.A.	MB, ChB	Albright and Wilson Ltd., London
Cooper	Mrs. H.	SRN, SCM, HV	Birmingham AHA
Cooper	Dr. M.I.	MB, BS, DPH	North Staffordshire HD
Cooper	Mrs.		Chelmsford HD
Cooperwaite	Miss A.L.	SRN	Fairmile Nursing Home, MCMF
Corcoran	Mrs. A.	SRN, SCM, HV	Bedfordshire AHA
Corkey	* Miss A.	BA	East Belfast and Castlereagh HD
Costello	L.		Eaton Laboratories, Surrey
Cotter	Mrs. E.	SRN, HV	West Sussex AHA
Couper	Miss S.	SRN	Hammersmith Hospital, London
Coverdale	* Mrs. I.M.		Warren Pearl House, MCMF
Cox	Miss S.J.	SRN	Weston Park Hospital, Sheffield
Cox	Miss S.J.	DN	Roding HD
Craig	Mrs. E.A.	SRN, SCM	St. Charles's Hospital, London
Craig	Mrs. N.A.	SRN, RFN, DN	Coventry AHA
Cran	* Mrs. F.	SEN	Domiciliary Nursing Service, MCMF
Crane	J.C.	SRN, DT	Suffolk AHA
Cripps	Mrs. D.	MSW	Horton Hospital, Banbury
Critchley	Miss J.A.	MCSP, SRP	London
Crosbie	R.J.	BA(Soc.Work)	Ipswich Hospital
Croston	Miss J.	SRN	Royal Cornwall Hospital, Truro
Culhane	Mrs. P.M.	MCSP	Colchester, Essex
Cullen	Mrs. E.	DN	Brent and Harrow AHA
Cunningham	Mrs. A.	SRN	St. Bartholomew's Hospital, London
Curran	Mrs. E.J.	SRN, SCM, DN	Leicestershire AHA
Currie	Miss R.H.	SRN, RNT	St. George's Hospital, London

Curtis	Miss E.S.	BSc	Ronkswood Hospital, Worcester
Curtis	Miss P.	FSR	Meyerstein Institute of Radiotherapy, London
Curtis-Prior	Dr. P.B.	BSc, PhD	Research Department, MCMF
Cussen	Sister C	SRN, ONC	St. Vincent's Orthopaedic Hospital, Middlesex
Cutler	* Dr. R.C.	MB, BS, LRCP, MRCS	London
Davey	Mrs. J.	Nursing Officer	Warren Pearl House, MCMF
Davidson	Dr. J.	MB, ChB(Edin)	General Accident Fire and Life Assurance Corporation
Davis	Mrs. F.B.	SRN, QN	Leicestershire AHA
Deakin	* Mrs. M.N.	SRN	Conrad House Nursing Home, MCMF
Dean	Dr. J.	MD, FRCP, FFCM	Medico-Social Research Board, Dublin
Degerland	* Mrs. S.E.	BTA, SRN, OHNC	Delta Rods (London) Ltd.
Densham	Miss A.M.	SRN, SCM, DN	Leicester AHA
Dexter	Mrs. S.A.	SRN	East Sussex AHA
Dickerson	Prof. J.W.	PhD,F.I.Biol.FIFST FRSH	University of Surrey
Dickie	Miss J.	Nursing Officer	DHSS, London
Dionne	Dr. L.		L'Hotel Dieu de Quebec, Canada
Diver	Miss M.		Medical Research Council, London
Dix	J.	SRN	Christie Hospital & Holt Radium Institute
Dodd	Miss V.A.	SRN	Cambridge AHA(T)
Dolton	Dr. W.D.	MA,MB,BChur,MRCS, LRCP,DPH,MFCM	Mersey RHA
Donaldson	* Dr. D.	MB,ChB,MRCP,MRCPath	Redhill General Hospital, Surrey
Donegan	Mrs. B.		Research Department, MCMF
Donnelly	Mrs. D.	Dip.PE,Cert.THE	Croydon AHA

Surname	Name	Qualifications	Affiliation
Dorrington	Miss J.	SRN, SCM, HV	Mid-Surrey HD
Douet	Miss S.M.	SRN, SCM, HV	Ealing, Hammersmith & Hounslow AHA
Dove	Miss I.M.	SRN, SCM, RCNT	St.Helier Hospital School of Nursing
Downie	*Miss P.A.	FCSP	London
Downie	W.A.	MB, ChB, FRCS Ed.	Victoria Hospital, Worksop
Downs	Mrs. E.H.	CSW	Manchester AHA(T)
Downton	Mrs. R.	SEN	Wessex Radiotherapy Centre
Doyle	Mrs. M.E.	SEN	St.Luke's Nursing Home, Sheffield
Draper	Miss P.	SRN, SCM, RNT	Chelmsford School of Nursing, Essex
Drumm	Mrs. M.M.	SRN, DN	Camden and Islington AHA
Drummond	Dr. J.	VRD, MB, ChB	Surrey AHA
Dudley	Mrs. R.C.	SRN, DN	Sheffield AHA
Dumigan	O.	SRN	Prince of Wales's Hospital, London
Dunkley	Miss A.M.	SRN, SCM, HV	Royal Marsden Hospital, London
Dyson	Miss G.	Nursing Officer	British Petroleum Co., Ltd., London
Ebling	Mrs. J.M.	SRN	Mount Hospital, Canterbury
Eddie	Miss H.		Research Department, MCMF
Edelstyn	Dr. G.	DMRT, MD, FFRCR	Eastern Area Health Board, Belfast
Edgerton	*Mrs. D.M.	SRN, DN	Harringay HD
Edwards	Mrs. M.	SRN, SCM, HV	Gloucestershire AHA
Edwards	Miss M.R.	MSW	Royal Gwent Hospital
Edwards	Mrs. N.		Research Department, MCMF
Edwards	Miss V.	SRN	B.U.P.A. Medical Centre, London
Efskind	Prof. L.		Norwegian Cancer Society, Oslo
Eldon	Miss A.M.	SRN, SCM	Cookridge Hospital, Leeds
Elkington	Miss J.		Imperial Cancer Research Fund, London
Elliott	Dr. B.A.	MD, FRCPath.	Miles Laboratories Ltd., Surrey
Ellis	Miss J.	SRN	Royal Marsden Hospital, London
Elsdon	Mrs. W.	SRN, SCM, DN, Dip.N.	Central Health Clinic, Corby

Elwood	Dr. W.J.	MB,BCL,BAO,MFCM,DPH	North Western RHA
Emerson	Mrs. J.	CQSW	City of Westminster
Evans	D.	RMN, SRN, RNT	School of Nursing, Hastings
Evans	Mrs. R.	SRN, SCM, DN	Lewisham HD
Feather	Mrs. S.	MSW	Radcliffe Infirmary, Oxford
Fennessy	Miss C.	Social Worker	City of Westminster
Fenton	Mrs. P.	Nursing Sister	St. Peter's Hospital, Surrey
Field	Dr. E.O.	MA,BM,BCh,DM,DMRD	Gallaher Ltd., London
Fielder	Miss M.		Redhill General Hospital, Surrey
Fincham	Miss P.J.	LCST	Hammersmith Hospital, London
Fish	Miss J.L.		Buckinghamshire AHA
Fisher	Mrs. E.M.	SRN, SCM, HV, DN	Westminster,Kensington & Chelsea AHA
Fisher	Dr. R.A.	MA,MRCS,LRCP,FFARCS	Christchurch Hospital, Dorset
Fisher	Miss W.	SRN, DN	Islington HD
Fitzgerald	Mrs. M.	Nursing Officer	Peterborough HD
Foley	* Miss M.A.	SRN	St.Joseph's Convalescent Home, Bournemouth
Forbes	Miss E.C.	SRN, SCM	St. Bartholomew's Hospital, London
Forbes	* Dr. W.	MD, PhD, FRCS Ed.	Scottish Home and Health Department
Ford	B.J.	SRN	Royal National Throat, Nose and Ear Hospital, London
Forder	B.A.	BSc, FPS, FRIC	Pfizer Ltd., Kent
Foster	Dr. H.L.	MB, ChB, DRCOG	St. Luke's Hospital, Surrey
Fowler	Mrs. H.C.	SRN, CMB,Dip.Health Ed.	Essex AHA
France	Mrs. M.	Nurse Tutor	Royal Infirmary, Huddersfield
Francis	Mrs. B.M.	SRN, ONC	Northampton HD
Francis	Miss S.B.	SRN	Coventry AHA
Freeman	Miss P.	SRN,	St. Bartholomew's Hospital, London
French	Miss D.E.	SRN, RCT	Withington Hospital, Manchester

French-Wollen	Mrs. J.	SRN	Wirral AHA
Friend	Mrs. M.F.	SRN, SCM, RMPA	London
Friend	Miss P.M.	CBE	DHSS, London
Furness	Miss B.	SRN, DN	Brookfields Hospital, Cambridge
Gaines	Miss B.W.	SRN, BTTA	Brompton Hospital, London
Galvin	Mrs. E.	Nurse Tutor	Royal Infirmary, Huddersfield
Gamage	Miss M.M.	SRN, SCM, QN, CTN, CHNT	King's College Hospital, London
Gamble	Mrs. A.	SRN	Booker Hospital, Buckinghamshire
Gardner	Dr. M.D.	MB, ChB, DPH	Lanarkshire Area Health Board
Garrett	Miss S.	MCSP	Royal Free Hospital, London
Gaskin	Mrs. J.M.	SRN, SCM, Dip.N, RNT	Coventry AHA
Geapin	Mrs. M.	SRN, DN	Greenwich and Bexley AHA
Gee	Miss E.A.	SRN, SCM	Bedfordshire AHA
Gent	* P.H.	MA, LL.B	Research Department, MCMF
George	Dr. A.M.	MB, BCh, DPH, MFCM	South Glamorgan AHA(T)
Gilbert	Mrs. B.E.	DSR	Devonshire AHA
Gill	Miss C.M.	SRN, SCM	Prince of Wales's Hospital, London
Gillard	Mrs. P.	SRN, DN, HV	Lewisham Hospital, London
Gillatt	Mrs. A.	SRN, SCM, HV, Dip.Soc.Sc.	Irish Cancer Society
Gillespie	Dr. A.V.	MB, DPH	Surrey AHA
Gillis	Dr. C.R.	MD, MFCM	Cancer Intelligence Unit, Glasgow
Gilliver	Miss M.I.	SRN	Royal Marsden Hospital, Surrey
Gilpin	* Rev. J.	Chaplain	Royal Infirmary, Sheffield
Gingell	Miss J.M.	SRN, SCM, ONC, RCT	Queen Elizabeth II Hospital, Herts.
Glanville	Miss E.	SRN, SCM	Royal South Hants Hospital, Southampton
Gledhill	* J.B.		Executive Committee, MCMF
Good	Miss A.M.	SEN	Hampshire AHA
Gooding	Miss N.A.	SRN, SCM	Ardenlea Nursing Home, MCMF

Gorbould	Miss M.S.	SRN	Royal National E.N.T. Hospital, London
Gordon	Miss M.		Research Department, MCMF
Gordon	Mrs. I.M.	SRN, RFN	Queen Victoria Memorial Home, Derby
Gough-Thomas	* Miss J.	MA	Executive Committee, MCMF
Gradwell	Mrs. R.E.	SRN	General Hospital, Plymouth
Gray	Miss J.	Dip.Soc.Stud. CQSW	City of Westminster
Gray	Miss L.J.	SRN, SCM, OND	University College Hospital, London
Grayston	Mrs. F.	SRN	Suffolk AHA
Greaves	Mrs. J.	SRN	Weston Park Hospital, Sheffield
Green	Mrs. E.M.	RGN, SCM	ITT Ltd., Kent
Green	Mrs. J.E.	SRN, DN	County Hospital, Hereford
Green	Mrs. M.	SRN	Manfield Hospital, Northampton
Green	Miss M.F.	BA(Hons)	Hither Green Hospital, London
Greenhalgh	Mrs. P.	SRN, DN	Bolton AHA
Greenway	* Lady		Executive Committee, MCMF
Gribbin	Brig. K.	MBE	Cancer Research Campaign
Griffin	Dr. G.V.	MB, BS, DPH, MFCM	Southend HD
Grimwade	Mrs. H.		Education/Welfare Committee, MCMF
Groom	Mrs. E.E.	SRN	RNIB Westcliff House
Groves	Miss M.	MSW	Royal Infirmary, Bristol
Gumuchian	Miss M.	BA	Christie Hospital & Holt Radium Inst.
Hackett	Miss R.A.	SRN	Warwickshire HD
Hague	Miss E.	SRN, SCM, DN	Mid-Surrey HD
Haig	Miss P.	SRN, SCM, HV	South-East Kent HD
Hale	Mrs. G.	Social Worker	Social Services Department, Coventry
Hall	Dr. C.E.	MB, ChB, DRCOG	DHSS, Belfast
Hall	R.F.	Social Worker	Social Services Dept., West Sussex
Halliday	Miss D.S.	SRN, SCM, HV	Bedfordshire AHA

Halliday		Mrs. M.	SRN, DN	Salford AHA(T)
Hamilton		Miss M.J.	SRN, SCM	Ashford Hospital, Middlesex
Hamilton		Mrs. S.S.	SRN	Royal Marsden Hospital, Surrey
Hammock		Mrs. S.	SRN, DN	Kent AHA
Hamon		Miss A.	SRN	St. George's Hospital, London
Hamson		Miss S.	SRN, SCM	Royal Nat. E.N.T. Hospital, London
Hancock		Mrs. A.C.	MCSP	Royal Marsden Hospital, Surrey
Hancock		Miss C.M.	BSc(Econ), SRN	Whipps Cross Hospital, London
Handby	*	J.G.		DHSS, London
Hansen		Dr. R.E.	MA,MB,BChir,DPH,FFCM	Cheltenham HD
Harden		Mrs. B.	MBAOT	Mount Vernon Hospital, Middlesex
Hardy		Mrs. P.D.	SRN	Hertfordshire AHA
Harmer		Dr. C.L.	MB,MRCP,FRCR	Royal Marsden Hospital, London
Harper		Miss P.M.	FSRTE	School of Radiography, Notts.
Harries	*	Mrs. M.L.	SRN	Charing Cross Hospital, London
Harris	*	R.G.	BSc, MIBiol.	Research Department, MCMF
Harris		Mrs. S.E.	SRN, ONC	St. George's Hospital, London
Harrison		Mrs. E.A.	MA, CQSW	Royal Infirmary, Bristol
Harvey		Mrs. D.V.	SRN	Luton and Dunstable Hospital
Harwood		Dr. H.F.		South-West Thames Reg.Cancer Council
Harwood		Mrs. S.	SRN,Dip.Soc.Studies	Queen Mary's Hospital, Sidcup
Haskell		Mrs. J.	Nursing Officer	School of Nursing, Oldchurch Hospital
Hatzigeorgiou		Miss K.M.	SRN	Royal Free Hospital, London
Hawkins		Miss E.J.	SRN	Prince of Wales's Hospital, London
Hawkins		Miss E.M.	SRN, HV, DN	Avon AHA
Hawthorne		Dr. V.M.	MD,FRCP(Glas),FFCM	University of Glasgow
Haxton		Miss M.M.	RGN, SCM	Greater Glasgow Health Board
Hayes		A.J.	BA, DSA	Wessex Oncology Service
Hayes		Miss M.P.	SRN	Charing Cross Hospital, London
Hayman		Miss O.H.	SRN	London Borough of Sutton

Haynes	Miss M.C.	SRN	Salisbury HD
Heald	* Lady	CBE	Executive Committee, MCMF
Heartfield	Rev. P.R.	Chaplain	Kent and Canterbury Hospital
Hedgman	* Mrs. M.	BSc(Pharm), MPS	Leo Laboratories Ltd., Middlesex
Henney	Mrs. D.P.	MSW	Whittington Hospital, London
Heyman	Dr. L.L.	BA, MB, BCh, BAO	Education/Welfare Committee, MCMF
Higgins	Miss M.I.	Nursing Officer	West Middlesex Hospital
Hill	Dr. E.B.	BSc,MB,ChB,DRCOG,MRCGP	Warren Pearl House, MCMF
Hill	Miss M.	Nursing Officer	Surrey AHA
Hines	Miss K.A.	SRN, SCM, DN	Cambridgeshire AHA(T)
Ho	Mrs. N.G.	SRN, SCM	West Middlesex Hospital
Hoadley	Mrs. D.M.	SRN, SCM, HV, MRSH	West Sussex AHA
Hocking	G.	SRN, DN, BTA	Great Yarmouth HD
Hodgson	R.W.	SRN, RNT, MCSP	Royal Nat. E.N.T. Hospital, London
Hogan	Mrs. M.	SRN,RFN,SCM,DN,HV	Nottinghamshire AHA(T)
Holland	Mrs. H.	SRN	Employment Medical Advisory Service
Holland	Miss M.	SRN, SCM, DN	Isle of Wight AHA
Hollins	Miss S.	MCSP	St. Mary's Hospital, London
Holmes	Dr. M.E.	MB, ChB	Sheffield AHA
Hooper	Dr. G.	MB, ChB, BSc	Eaton Laboratories, Surrey
Horan	Miss M.A.	SRN	Kensington,Chelsea & Westminster AHA
Hosker	Miss C.A.	SRN SCM	St. George's Hospital, London
Howes	Miss P.	SRN	Royal Marsden Hospital, London
Howman	Mrs. B.	SRN	St. James's Hospital, London
Hoy	Miss J.	DSR(T)	Hammersmith Hospital, London
Hubbard	Mrs. M.E.	SRN	Royal South Hants Hospital
Hudson	Mrs. A.	DSR(T)	United Oxford Hospitals
Hudson-Williams	Mrs. J.		Conrad House Nursing Home, MCMF
Hughes	Mrs. C.M.	Nursing Officer	Worcester HD
Hughes	Dr. J.P.	TD, MD, DPH	Albright and Wilson Ltd., London

Hunnybun		Dr. J.	MB, BS, DRCOG	Health Centre, Caterham, Surrey
Hunt		Miss P.J.	SRN	Royal Infirmary, Bristol
Hurst	*	Miss A.G.	SRN, CMB(PtI)	St. Thomas's Hospital, London
Hurst		Miss J.M.	SRN, SCM	Buchanan Hospital, Sussex
Hutchison		Dr. J.	MB, ChB	Marks and Spencer Ltd., London
Inglis		Mrs. M.B.	Inst.Almoner	City of Westminster
Ironside		Dr. D.N.	MB,ChB,DPH,MFCM	Tonbridge HD
Jackson	*	Dr. D.	MD	Abbott Laboratories Ltd., Kent
Jackson		Miss M.M.		Royal Free Hospital, London
James		Dr. M.L.	MB, BCh, BSc	Holme Tower Nursing Home, MCMF
James		Miss S.A.	SRN	Charing Cross Hospital, London
Jansen		Mrs. J.	AAPSW	Raigmore Hospital, Inverness
Jarema	*	Dr. R.S.	MB, ChB	St. John of God Hospital, Yorkshire
Jarman		Miss F.M.	SRN, HV, DN	Islington HD
Jeal	*	S.C.	HND	Research Department, MCMF
Jefferson		Miss M.	SRN, RSCN	Mount Vernon Hospital, Middlesex
Jeffreson		Mrs. H.	MCSP	Mount Vernon Hospital, Middlesex
Jenkins		Miss D.L.	BSc, AIMSW	Bedford Hospital
Jenner		Mrs. M.	BSc	Research Department, MCMF
John		Miss B.M.	SRN, SCM, RCNT	University Hospital of Wales
John		Mrs. V.M.	SRN	University Hospital of Wales
Johnson		Mrs. A.E.	SRN, DN	Kent AHA
Johnson		Miss D.	SRN, HV	Hastings HD
Jones		G.V.	SRN, RMN	Knowle Hospital, Hampshire
Jones		Mrs. M.	SRN, QN	Preston HD
Jones		Mrs. P.A.	HV	Buckinghamshire AHA
Jones		Miss P.D.	O.St.J, SRN, SCM	DHSS, Welsh Office
Jones		Miss S.J.	SRN, SCM	Wirral AHA

Surname	Name	Qualifications	Institution
Jordan	Miss D.N.	SRN	Gloucester HD
Jordan	Mrs. E.F.	SRN, RCNT	Cuckfield and Crawley HD
Jordan	Mrs. J.A.	SRN, RCNT, CMB(PtI)	Wycombe General Hospital, Bucks.
Jovanovic	Mrs. M.	SRN	Buckinghamshire AHA
Kanterovitz	Rabbi M.	BA, AMWI	General Infirmary, Leeds
Kapadia	Mrs. B.	SRN, DN	Ashford Hospital, Middlesex
Keenan	Miss J.A.	SRN, SCM, ICUCert.	The London Clinic
Kelly	Mrs. K.M.	SRN	Downside Hospital, Sussex
Kelly	* Miss M.B.	RGN, SCM	Ninewells Hospital, Dundee
Kemp	Mrs. C.S.	SRN	Essex AHA
Kenny	A.W.	MA,BSc,C.Chem,FRIC	Department of the Environment,London
Kernighan	Mrs. A.	SRN,RSCN,CMB(PtI)	United Liverpool Hospitals
Kevill	Miss P.J.	SRN, SCM	Manchester AHA(T)
Khan	Miss A.	SRN	Harringay HD
Khatir	Mrs. I.K.		Royal Free Hospital, London
King	N.G.	SRN, ONC, DN	South Derbyshire HD
King-Wilkinson	Miss B.J.	SRN, RCT	St. Thomas's Hospital, London
Kinnier Wilson	Dr. L.M.	MA, BM, BCh.	Research Department, MCMF
Kinsella	B.A.	SRN, DN	Hastings HD
Kirkland	Mrs. I.F.	RFN, SRN, SCM	Prince of Wales's Hospital, London
Klar	Mrs. A.B.	AIMSW	Department of Social Services,London
Klar	S.	MPS	St. Charles's Hospital, London
Knibbs	Mrs. E.M.	SRN, CMB, DN	Greenwich and Bexley AHA
Knight	Mrs. C.A.	SRN,ONC,DN,RCNT	School of Nursing, Nottingham
Knowles	Mrs. A.P.	SRN, SCM	General Hospital, Birmingham
Lalor	* Miss S.J.	BSc.	Research Department, MCMF
Lambie	Mrs. J.	Staff Nurse	St. William's Hospital, Rochester
Lance	Mrs. G.A.	SRN	Hillingdon AHA

Lang	Miss C.	SRN, RCNT	Royal Marsden Hospital, London
Lang	Mrs. M.	MA(Hons),Dip.Soc.Adm.	Royal Infirmary, Dundee
Law	Miss D.	MCSP	Chest Hospital, London
Lawrence	Miss J.	SRN, SCM	Churchill Hospital, Oxford
Lawrence	Mrs. J.M.	SRN,RFN,Dip.N(Lond)	Derbyshire AHA
Lawrie	Miss M.	SRN	Royal Marsden Hospital, Surrey
Lawson	*Mrs. D.	SRN, DN	Buckinghamshire AHA
Laxton	Mrs. W.	Social Worker	Leicestershire C.C.
Leaver	Dr. J.M.	MB, BS	City and Hackney HD
Lee	P.N.	MA	Tobacco Research Council, London
Le Gassick	Miss J.	SRN, SCM	Hillingdon Hospital, Middlesex
Lerch	Mrs. M.	SRN, SCM	Wiltshire AHA
Lester	Miss B.	SRN	South London Hospital
Linford	H.G.	SRN, DN	Ipswich HD
Ling	Miss H.K.	Chaplain	Royal Free Hospital, London
Lister	Rev. G.H.	DSR, SRR	Leeds Infirmary, Yorkshire
Litchfield	Mrs. F.B.	SRN, CMB, OHNC	London
Lloyd	Mrs. E.	SRN	Courage and Eastern Ltd., London
Lloyd-Owen	Miss J.	SRN	BUPA Medical Centre, London
Lobb	Miss D.	FSR(T),Dip.Soc.Stud.	Royal Cornwall Hospital, Truro
Lochhead	Miss J.	MA, RGN, RNT	Royal Free Hospital, London
Logan	Miss W.	SRN	Scottish Home & Health Department
Loman	H.T.	SRN, RCNT	St. Ann's Hospital, London
Loveday	Miss O.M.	BA	St.Mary's School of Nursing, London
Lovegreen	Miss A.	MB, BAO, BCh.	Nightingale School of Nursing,London
Lowry	Dr. M.	MB, DMRT, FRCR	Ballymena Health Centre, N. Ireland
Lynch	Dr. G.A.		Eastern Health & Social Services Board, Northern Ireland
Lyons	Dr. J.	MB,ChB,MRCS,LRCP,DPH, FFCM	Devon AHA

Lyons	Mrs. M.B.		West Middlesex Hospital
McAuley	P.	BSc(Hons)	Ulster Cancer Foundation
McAuliffe	Miss J.M.	Nursing Officer	Royal Marsden Hospital, London
McBeath	Mrs. C.M.	RGN, DN	Lothian Health Board
McBride	Miss J.	MCSP	Lodge Road Clinic, Surrey
McCartie	Dr. K.M.	MRCS,LRCP,DRCOG	Douglas McMillen Home, Staffs
MacDonald	* Dr. D.	MB, ChB	Hill of Tarvit Nursing Home, MCMF
McGarrigle	Miss M.	RGN, SCM	Greater Glasgow Health Board
McGee	Miss K.	SRN, SCM	Royal Nat.Throat,Nose & Ear Hospital
McIlrath	Dr. R.A.	MB	Beaconfield Nursing Home, MCMF
McInnes	Mrs.	SRN, DN	East Dorset Health District
McKeown	Miss T.B.	SRN	Eastern Health Board, Belfast
Mackie	* Dr. E.D.	MB,ChB,DPH,MFCM	Yorkshire RHA
MacLean	Miss A.	SRN	St. Bartholomew's Hospital, London
McLean	Dr. A.	Grad.RIC,MSc,PhD	Research Department, MCMF
McLeod	G.K.		Imperial Cancer Research Fund,London
MacLeod	Mrs. M.	Social Worker	Oldchurch Hospital, Essex
MacMaster	Mrs. M.M.	SRN, DN	Bedfordshire AHA
McNab	Miss M.E.	SRN, STD, RNT	Luton and Dunstable Hospital
McNelly	Mrs. D.M.	LCST	Royal Marsden Hospital, Surrey
MacPherson	Dr. M.	MB, ChB, DA	Medical Research Council, London
MacRae	Dr. J.H.	MB, ChB	London
McSorley	Mrs. S.C.	SRN	Gulson Hospital, Coventry
McWade	Mrs. L.G.	SRN, SCM, HV	Maternity Hospital, Ipswich
Macey	Mrs. R.	Social Worker	Social Services Dept., West Sussex
Maddever	Miss R.M.	SRN, SCM, RNT	Plymouth HD
Magee	Mrs. R.A.	MSW	North Middlesex Hospital
Maguire	Miss C.	SRN	Hillingdon Hospital, Middlesex
Mahony	D.	SRN, RMN, DN	East Birmingham Hospital

Mahood	Mrs. P.M.	SRN	West Birmingham HD
Makins	Miss J.	SRN	Eastbourne HD
Malcolm-Smith	Mrs. Y.	SRN, CMB(PtI)	Mount Hospital, Canterbury
Maldonado	Mrs. P.E.	Nurse Tutor	School of Nursing, Hammersmith Hospital
Malthouse	Miss M.S.	MBAOT	Mount Vernon Hospital, Middlesex
Manser	Miss C.A.	SRN, HV, CQSW	Queen Elizabeth Hospital, Birmingham
Mantzalos	Miss S.		Royal Free Hospital, London
Marchant	Mrs. J.		Chelmsford HD
Markby	Miss R.	SRN, SCM	St. Bartholomew's Hospital, London
Marshall	Miss L.	BA(Soc.Admin)	The London Hospital
Marshall	Miss N.		Research Department, MCMF
Martin	Mrs. C.	Social Worker	Harold Wood Hospital, Essex
Mathews	Mrs. J.	SRN, SCM, HV	Houth East Kent HD
Matthew	Miss E.	MSW	Mildmay Mission Hospital
Matthews	Miss E.	SRN	Lambeth Hospital, London
Mattock	Mrs. C.M.	SRN	Abingdon Hospital, Oxfordshire
Maya	Mrs. M.L.	SRN, SCM, DN	Wiltshire AHA
Meier	Miss J.	SRN, RCNT	School of Nursing, St. Mary's Hospital, London
Melvin	Mrs. S.W.	Nursing Officer	Royal Infirmary, Dumfries
Metcalfe	Miss S.		Research Department, MCMF
Meyer	Dr. M.	MB, BS	British Broadcasting Corp., London
Michie	Miss H.R.		Research Department, MCMF
Milburn	Miss P.M.	SRN	North Middlesex Hospital
Millar	Dr. I.B.	MD,BCh,BAO,DPH,MFCM	Greenwich HD
Millar	Mrs. M.T.	SRN, RMN	DHSS, Belfast
Miller	Miss W.E.	SRN, RSCN	St. George's Hospital, London
Mills	Miss J.	BA(Hons), M.Phil.	Research Department, MCMF
Mills	Miss R.	TDSRT	School of Radiotherapy, Middlesex Hospital

Missenden	Mrs. M.	SRN, SCM	Royal Berkshire Hospital
Mitchell	Mrs. A.	Social Worker	Royal Marsden Hospital, Surrey
Mitchell	Miss P.R.	BA, AIMSW	General Hospital, Plymouth
Mitchell	Miss S.M.	SRN	Royal Marsden Hospital, London
Moffitt	Miss J.L.	SRN, OHNC	ITT(U.K.) Ltd., London
Mogg	Sister P.	SRN	Christchurch Hospital, Dorset
Mollitt	Mrs. H.W.	SRN, RSON	Cookridge Hospital, Leeds
Moody	Mrs. L.	SRN	Warren Pearl Nursing Home, MCMF
Morek	Miss M.	SRN	Hammersmith Hospital, London
Morris	Miss A.S.		Imperial Cancer Research Fund, London
Morris	Mrs. W.A.	SRN, ONC	Cleveland AHA
Moss	Miss J.E.	SRN, SCM, DN, HV	Preston Hall Hospital, Kent
Mowbray	Mrs. M.L.	MCSP	Maida Vale Hospital, London
Munday	Miss M.A.	SRN	General Hospital, Bedford
Murphy	A.	SRN, RMN	Harold Wood Hospital, Essex
Murray	Miss M.		Warren Pearl Nursing Home, MCMF
Miter	Mrs. R.	SRN, DN	Surrey AHA
Neagle	Miss J.I.	SRN, QN	Dorset AHA
Neale	Miss E.	Social Worker	Worthing Hospital, Sussex
Neave	Mrs. J.I.	MA, SRN, RSCN	General Hospital, Cheltenham
Neeve	Miss E.	SRN	St. Ann's Hospital, London
Nellen	Mrs. F.		Women's Nat.Cancer Control Campaign
Nelson Bowgett	Mrs. G.M.	FSSCh, ASSF, ACh.	Bispham, Lancashire
Nevill	Mrs. G.E.	SRN	Royal Marsden Hospital, London
Newman	Rev.Br.M.	SRN,Dip.N(Pt A)	St. Cuthbert's Hospital, Co. Durham
Newson	Miss D.		Research Department, MCMF
Nicol	Dr. W.	Medical Officer	Birmingham AHA(T)
Nobbs	B.R.	SRN, RMN, RNT	Norwich HD
Northfield	Dr. R.	MB, BS, DA, DJH	British Airways, London

Surname	Name	Qualifications	Institution
Oakes	* Mrs. M.	BSc, CQSW, Dip.App. Soc.Studies	The London Hospital
O'Brien	Mrs. P.		Gerard's Cross, Buckinghamshire
O'Dwyer	Miss M.E.	SRN, SCM, HV	Dorset AHA
O'Flynn	Mrs. M.P.	SRN	Dartford and Gravesend HD
Ojobode	J.O.	DSRR	University Teaching Hospital, Lagos
Okane	Mrs. E.	SRN	Kent AHA
Orr	Mrs. J.M.	SRN, SCM, RMT	District Hospital, Basingstoke
Osborne	* Miss J.M.	SRN, CMB(PtI), NNEB	Betts & Co., Ltd., Colchester
Osman	Miss V.M.	SRN, SCM	Wessex Radiotherapy Centre
Ospala	Miss M.	MSW	Royal National Orthopaedic Hospital
Owen	J.W.	MA	St. Thomas's HD
Owen	Dr. R.	MB, ChB, DMJ, DIH, LRIC	Employment Medical Advisory Service
Ower	Dr. D.C.	Principal M.O.	DHSS, London
Owst	Miss C.	SRN, SCM, HV	Brighton HD
Pace	Mrs. P.I.	MSW	Social Services Department, Suffolk
Paddon	Mrs. D.E.	SRN	Royal Free Hospital, London
Page	Miss J.A.	DSRT	Devonshire AHA
Palmer	Mrs. B.	SRN, HV	Berkshire AHA
Palmer	Miss B.E.	SRN, RSCN	East Dorset HD
Pantling	Miss P.P.	SRN, BTA	Canterbury and Thanet HD
Papp	Mrs. J.	SRN	Royal Marsden Hospital, London
Pardey	E.T.	SRN, RMN, RMT	Banstead Hospital, Surrey
Pardy	Mrs. I.	SRN, ONC, DN	Ashford Hospital, Middlesex
Park	Miss J.	DSRT	Hammersmith Hospital, London
Parken	Dr. D.S.	MB, BS, MRCS, LRCP, DCH, DPH, MFCM	Lancashire AHA
Parker	Miss L.M.	Social Worker	The London Hospital
Parnell	Miss J.W.	SRN, SCM, HV, DN	Queen's Nursing Institute, London

Surname	Name	Qualifications	Affiliation
Parry-Davies	* Mrs. S.	MSW	Royal Free Hospital, London
Parslow	Miss K.	SRN, SCM, HV, DN	Polegate, Sussex
Parsons	Mrs. B.	SRN, KRN	Bedfordshire AHA
Parsons	H.M.	FRCS	General Hospital, Croydon
Parsons	Mrs. P.	SEN, DN	Isle of Wight AHA
Parsons	Miss A.		Executive Committee, MCMF
Paterson	Dr. T.G.	MB, ChB	Railway Convalescent Homes, Margate
Paterson	Miss C.	Nursing Officer	St. Peter's Hospital, Surrey
Patrick	Mrs. M.H.	SRN, DN, CMB(PtI)	Hertfordshire AHA
Patterson	* Mrs. D.C.	HNC	Research Department, MCMF
Payne	* Mrs. D.P.		Research Department, MCMF
Payne	Mrs. H.H.		Dorset AHA
Payne	Dr. L.R.	SRN	Employment Medical Advisory Service
Pearce	Mrs. J.M.	MB, ChB	Ashford Hospital, Middlesex
Peart	Miss I	SRN	Mid-Surrey HD
Peatfield	G.R.	SRN, SCM, DM	General Hospital, Bedford
Penney	* Miss A.	MChir, FRCS	DHSS, London
Penney	Dr. J.P.	OBE, SRN, SCM, HV	ITT(UK) Ltd., Kent
Perry	Mrs. O.P.	MB, ChB	Mid-Staffordshire HD
Phillips	Mrs. E.A.	SRN	Kent AHA
Phillips	Miss M.E.	SRN, DN	School of Nursing, Hammersmith Hospital
Pickering	* Mrs. M.	SRN, RSCN, RNT	Enfield HD
Pierce	Miss I	SRN, DN	Nightingale School of Nursing, London
Pigott	Miss M.	SNO(Tutor)	Addenbrooke's Hospital, Cambridge
Piltrow	Miss D.A.	SRN	Lewisham HD
Pilling	* Mrs. E.F.	SRN, DN	Buckinghamshire AHA
Pine	Dr. I.M.	SRN, DN	Dept. of Community Health, Portsmouth
Pinkerton	Dr. M.	MB, BS, DPH, MFCP	Marks and Spencer Ltd., London
Pinkney	Mrs. F.	MB, BCh, DPH, FRSH, FRIPHH	Poole Hospital, Cleveland
Pinnock	Miss M.	SRN, QN	Research Department, MCMF

Politi	Mrs. J.	SRN, RNT	School of Nursing, St. George's Hospital, London
Pollock	Dr. G.T.	MB, ChB, MFCM, DPH	Coventry AHA
Pommells	Mrs. E.M.	SRN	St. Ann's Hospital, London
Poole	Miss S.A.	SRN, SCM	Essex AHA
Pooley	Miss M.C.	SRN	County Hospital, Dorchester
Poston	J.W.	B.Pharm., MPS	Wellcome Foundation Ltd., Herts.
Potter	Mrs. J.	Social Worker	Charing Cross Hospital, London
Poulson	Miss S.	SRN, SCM	The London Hospital
Povey	Dr. W.P.	MRCS, LRCP, MFCM, DPH, DRCOG	Manchester AHA(T)
Powell	Mrs. A.M.	BA(Soc.Sc), DASS, CQSW	Cheshire County Council
Powell	R.	SRN	Dorset AHA
Prentice	D.E.	MA, Vet.MB, MVSc, MRCVS	Huntingdon Research Centre
Priestnall	Miss S.	SRN	St. Luke's Nursing Home, London
Prior	Miss E.	SRN, SCM, DN	Wiltshire AHA
Proctor	Miss J.E.	MCSP	London
Proudlove	Miss K.	SRN, OND	Royal Hospital, Wolverhampton
Prynn	Mrs. B.	Social Worker	Brook General Hospital, London
Pullen	Miss E.A.	SRN, ONC, RCNT, CMB(PtI)	University College Hospital, London
Quartly	Mrs. J.M.	SRN, SCM, HV	Cardinal Road Clinic, Middlesex
Quayle	Miss B.	SRN, SCM	United Oxford Hospita⁻s
Quinnell	* Mrs. L.G.	SRN	Wessex Radiotherapy Centre
Rae	Mrs. S.J.	SRN	Lambeth, Southwark & Lewisham AHA
Raeburn	Mrs. P.	RGN	Belvedere Hospital, Glasgow
Raggett	Mrs. M.T.	SRN, SCM	British Petroleum Co., Ltd., London
Raha	Mrs. M.W.	SRN	Royal National E.N.T. Hospital, London
Rasbridge	* Mrs. M.R.	FIMLS	Leo Laboratories Ltd., Middlesex

Surname	Name	Qualifications	Institution
Rashley	Miss N.M.	SRN	Royal Infirmary, Bristol
Raven	* Dame Kathleen	DBE, SRN, SCM	Wing, Bedfordshire
Rayner	Miss L.	Chaplain	Addenbrookes Hospital, Cambridge
Rea	Miss L.V.	SRN, RMN	St. Bartholomew's Hospital, London
Redfern	* Mrs. J.L.	MIMSW	Epsom District Hospital, Surrey
Reed	Mrs. J.		Research Department, MCMF
Reeder	Mrs. E.	Nursing Officer	St. William's Hospital, Kent
Reeves	Miss K.E.	SRN	Gordon Hospital, London
Rehan	Miss M.J.	CQSW	Queen Elizabeth Hospital, Birmingham
Reid	Mrs. F.M.	STN, RNT	School of Nursing, Bedford
Rendle	Miss M.A.	SEN	Cheltenham Group Hospitals
Reynolds	Mrs. P.M.	Social Worker	General Hospital, Kettering
Rice	Mrs. A.	SRN	Humberside AHA
Richards	Dr. D.P.	MB,BS,DCH,DPH,MFCM	Lewisham HD
Riches	* Miss E.	SRN, SCM	St. Bartholomew's Hospital, London
Richmond	Dr. H.A.	MB, ChB	Strathclyde House Nursing Home, MCMF
Richter	Miss A.	SRN	BUPA Medical Centre, London
Rivers	Mrs. J.	Occupational Therapist	Connaught Hospital, London
Rix	Mrs. J.	MSW	Royal Nat.Orthopaedic Hospital,London
Roberts	Miss A.C.	SRN, SCM	Whittington Hospital, London
Roberts	Miss J.H.	SRN	University College Hospital, London
Roberts	Miss M.	BSc	Research Department, MCMF
Roberts	Dr. P.A.	MB, BS	London
Robertshaw	Mrs. M.		Research Department, MCMF
Robertson	* Mrs. D.M.	MSW	Charing Cross Hospital, London
Robertson	Miss J.W.	SRN, HV	Avon AHA
Robins	Miss W.	SRN	Dudley Road Hospital, Birmingham
Robinson	* Mrs. D.	CQSW	Social Services Department, Coventry
Robinson	Miss J.	SRN	Hammersmith Hospital, London

Robinson	Miss M.J.	SRN, SCM, HV	General Hospital, Birmingham
Robinson	Mrs. M.J.	Social Worker	Social Services Department, Essex
Robinson	* S/Ldr. T.B.	OBE, FCIS	Founder Secretary, MCMF
Robson	Dr. D.R.	PhD	Parke, Davis and Company, Gwent
Robson	Miss S.M.	DSRT	Hammersmith Hospital, London
Rockliff	Miss M.	BSc, SRN	University of Birmingham
Rohlehr	Miss A.	HV	Hastings HD
Rondi	Mrs. G.	BSc(Soc.Studies)	Lewisham Hospital, London
Rosbottom	Miss J.	SRN	Royal Marsden Hospital, Surrey
Rose	Mrs. E.D.	MCSP	Westminster Hospital, London
Rosevink	Miss M.	DSR	United Hospitals, Bristol
Round	Miss J.A.	SRN	St. Luke's Hospital, Surrey
Rowark	Mrs. L.	SRN	Berkshire AHA
Rowdon	Mrs. M.	SEN	Dartford and Gravesend HD
Rowe	* Miss D.	SRN	Royal Free Hospital, London
Rowe	* Dr. J.J.	BSc,PhD,Grad.RIC	Research Department, MCMF
Rowlands	* Mrs. S.	CQSW	City of Westminster
Rudd	Mrs. J.M.	SRN	Royal Infirmary, Leicester
Rush	Miss M.E.	DSRT	North Middlesex Hospital
Rushton	Miss L.M.		St.John & Red Cross Society, London
Russell	Sister M.	SEN	St.Joseph's Convalescent Home, Bournemouth
Russell	Mrs. P.J.	SRN, RCNT	Hammersmith Hospital, London
Ruttley	Mrs. J.F.	SEN, CQSW	Freedom Fields Hospital
Sadleir	T.R.		Cancer Research Campaign, London
Saffery	* Miss P.	SRN	Harestone Nursing Home, MCMF
Samuels	Miss M.W.	SRN, SCM, DTN	Hereford and Worcester AHA
Sanderson	Dr. R.L.	MB, ChB, MRCGP	Ashby de la Zouche
Scarlett	Miss A.	SEN	Charing Cross Hospital, London

Schmidt	Mrs. M.C.	Nursing Officer	King's HD
Schofield	Miss G.F.	SRN, SCM, DN	South West Thame RHA
Scott	Miss M.L.	SRN, SCM	Moyle Hospital, Northern Ireland
Scott	Mrs. V.J.	SRN, SCM	General Hospital, Poole
Scruby	Miss I.V.	SRN, HV	Greenwich and Bexley AHA
Seach	Mrs. A.F.	SRN, QN	Southend HD
Seale	Mrs. R.	SRN, SCM, HV	Kingston and Richmond AHA
Seaman	Mrs. M.J.	SRN	East Dorset HD
Seaton-Sykes	* Mrs. C.M.	SRN	Royal United Hospitals, Bath
Self	C.D.		Tower Hamlets AHA
Seppelt	Dr. I.	MA,MB,BChir,DPH,MFCM	Barnet AHA
Seymour	H.C.	BSc, Dip.Ed.	British Cancer Council
Shaw	Mrs. B.E.	SEN	Hampshire AHA
Shaw	H.J.	VRD, MA, FRCS	Royal Marsden Hospital, London
Shaw	Mrs. I.	SRN, CMB(PtI)	Royal South Hants Hospital,Southampton
Shaw	* N.M.	MPS	Lundbeck Ltd., Luton
Sheldon	Miss E.M.	BA(Hons)	Walton Hospital, Liverpool
Sheldrake	Miss P.A.	Nursing Officer	Selly Oak Hospital
Sherwood	Mrs. M.	DN	Central Middlesex Hospital
Shewan	Miss G.M.	SRN, SCM	Cookbridge Hospital, Leeds
Silcox	* Miss J.J.	BSc, LIBiol.	Research Department, MCMF
Simpson	Dr. I.G.	MB,ChB,Dip.Soc.Med.	Grampian Health Board, Scotland
Sims	Mrs. J.	SRN, RCNT	West Roding School of Nursing, London
Sims	Dr. P.A.	MSc,MB,BS,BDS	Newham HD
Sinclair	N.A.	DSRT	Hammersmith Hospital, London
Singh	Sister M.	SRN, SCM	Maternity Hospital, Ipswich
Siviter	Mrs. S.E.	SRN	Sandwell AHA
Skinner	Mrs. B.P.	SRN, DN	Medway HD
Slattery	Mrs. M.A.	BA(Hons), MSW	Radcliffe Infirmary, Oxford
Sleigh	Mrs. S.J.	SRN, RCT	Kingston-upon-Thames, Surrey

Surname	Name	Qualifications	Affiliation
Smethurst	* Dr. M.	BSc, PhD, M.I.Biol.	Research Department, MCMF
Smith	Mrs. A.M.		Research Department, MCMF
Smith	C.R.	SRN, RMN	Ealing, Hammersmith & Hounslow AHA
Smith	Dr. D.L.		Employment Medical Advisory Service
Smith	Mrs. I.J.	SRN	Oldchurch Hospital, Essex
Smith	* J.P.	BSc(Soc),DER,SRN,RNT, BTA Cert.	Central Middlesex Hospital, London
Smith	Miss M.	SRN	West Berkshire HD
Smith	Miss M.	SRN, SCM	Royal Infirmary, Bristol
Smith	* Mrs. N.	BSc(Hons)	Research Department, MCMF
Snelling	Dr. M.R.	OBE,MRCS,LRCP,FRCP	Lloyds Bank Ltd., London
Soloff	Dr. N.		Northamptonshire AHA
Somervell	Mrs. K.M.	AIMSW	Walsall Guild of Voluntary Service
Specterman	Miss E.	SRN, CMB(PtI)	Southend HD
Spice	Mrs. J.	SRN	Buchanan Hospital, Sussex
Spinak	Mrs. A.	SRN	Hastings HD
Springate	P.A.	SRN, OHNC	Queen Mary's Hospital, Kent
Spry	Miss E.	SRN, SCM, HV	Lewisham HD
Standish	Mrs. B.M.	SRN, CMB(PtI)	Horton General Hospital, Oxfordshire
Stanning	Miss R.	MA	Hackney Hospital, London
Staton	Miss M.C.	SRN, SCM, AAPSW	Westminster City Council
Staunton	M.D.	MCh, FRCS	Executive Committee, MCMF
Steele	Miss T.	Social Worker	West Sussex County Council
Stepheni	Rev. F.W.	Chaplain	Addenbrookes Hospital, Cambridge
Stephens	Miss M.E.	SEN	Middlesex Hospital, London
Stephenson	Mrs. J.	MBE, SRN, SCM, DN, HV	Humberside AHA
Stewart	* Miss A.T.	RGN, SCM	Tidcombe Hall Nursing Home, MCMF
Stewart	Mrs. K.	SRN, RCNT	School of Nursing, Sheffield
Stewart	Dr. M.	MB, ChB	Marks and Spencer, Ltd., London
Stillwell	Dr. J.M.	MRCS, LRCP	Buckinghamshire AHA

Stone	Miss M.M.	SRN, SCM	Medical Research Council, London
Storey	Mrs. D.E.	SRN	Weston Park Hospital, Sheffield
Storti	Miss C.	SRN, RMN	St. Charles's Hospital, London
Stubbs	Mrs. M.	SRN, RCNT	Queen Mary's Hospital, Kent
Sutcliffe	* Mrs. M.	SRN, RCNT	School of Nursing, Rochdale
Sutherland	Miss A.G.	SRN, SCM	Stratholyde Nursing Home, MCMF
Sutton	Mrs. A.	SRN, SCM, DN	Coventry AHA
Swain	Mrs. P.	Clinical Teacher	Windsor School of Nursing, Berkshire
Swash	J.I.	MRSH	Spencer (Surgical Supplies)Ltd.Oxford
Sydserff	Miss M.G.	RGN, SCM	Hillingdon Hospital, Middlesex
Sykes	Mrs. R.M.	SRN	General Hospital, Northampton
Tart	Mrs. J.	SRN	Royal Infirmary, Leicester
Tate	H.		Medical Research Council, London
Taylor	Miss B.M.	SRN, OHNC, SCM	ITT(UK) Ltd., London
Taylor	Miss F.B.	FSR	North Middlesex Hospital
Taylor	Dr. G.C.		S.-W. Thames Regional Cancer Council
Taylor	Mrs. M.	Social Worker	Barking Hospital, Essex
Taylor	Miss P.	SRN, SCM, DN	Cornwall and Isles of Scilly AHA
Teare	* Mrs. J.W.	SRN, DN	Bromley AHA
Thomas	Mrs. J.D.	SRN, CMB(PtI)	St. Mary's Hospital, London
Thomas	Miss J.E.	BSc	Health Education Council, London
Thompson	Mrs. B.	SRN	Great Yarmouth and Waveney HD
Thompson	Mrs. J.		Research Department, MCMF
Thompson	Miss L.	BSc	University of Manchester
Thornley	Mrs.	SRN, DN	East Dorset HD
Timmins	Miss N.	SRN	Solihull Hospital, Warwickshire
Tod	Dr. E.D.	JP, MB, ChB, MRCGP	Kingston, Surrey
Todd	* G.F.	OBE	S.-W. Thames Regional Cancer Council
Toff	Mrs. J.	MSW	Royal Nat. Orthopaedic Hospital,London

Tomlinson	Mrs. M.	Nursing Officer	South Tees HD
Toone	* Mrs. M.	SRN	St. James's Hospital, London
Torrance-Allen	Dr. L.	MD, ChB, FRCOG	Woolwich Group of Hospitals
Torrie	Dr. E.C.	MD, DPH	Northern Health Board, N. Ireland
Tregoning	Miss R.F.	SRN	Prince of Wales's Hospital, London
Tripptree	* Mrs. J.L.	SRN, NNEB, DN	Kingston and Richmond AHA
Troy	Dr. J.J.	MB, BCh.	Camden and Islington AHA(T)
Tucker	Mrs.	BSc(Soc.)	Social Services Department, Hillingdon
Tucker	Mrs. N.R.	SRN	Addenbrookes Hospital, Cambridge
Turner	Miss M.E.	SRN, SCM, HV	Ealing,Hammersmith & Hounslow AHA(T)
Turpin	R.J.	SRN, DN	Barking HD
Upton	* Mrs. D.		Research Department, MCMF
Urquhart	Miss C.M.	BSc.	Research Department, MCMF
Vatcher	* A.R.	SRN, RNT, OStJ	Cambridgeshire AHA(T)
Vega	Dr. E.J.	MB, ChB, DLO	Newland Health Centre, Lincoln
Vincent	Miss J.A.	SRN, SCM	Prince of Wales's Hospital, London
Wade	Dr. H.E.	BA, PhD	Microbiological Research Establishment, Wiltshire
Wagstaffe	Mrs. P.	SRN	Wessex Radiotherapy Centre
Walji	Miss F.	SRN	Weston Park Hospital, Sheffield
Walker	Mrs. J.	SRN, SCM, DN	Bedfordshire AHA
Wall	Miss C.	SRN, DHSA	DHSS, London
Wallace	Miss R.H.	SRN	St. Bartholomew's Hospital, London
Walley	* Miss F.I.	SRN, DN	Mid-Staffordshire HD
Wallis	Dr. R.W.	MB,BS,MRCS,LRCP,DRCOG, MRCGP	Horncastle, Lincolnshire
Walters	Mrs. J.	BA, AMIMSW	Kingston-upon-Thames Hospital, Surrey

Walton	Mrs. B.L.	DSRT	Leicester AHA(T)
Walton	Mrs. D.K.	SRN, RMN, DN	Medway HD
Ward	Mrs. M.	SRN, SCM, RNCT	Hammersmith Hospital, London
Ward	Mrs. M.A.	SRN	Wiltshire AHA
Wares	Miss E.W.	RFN, SRN, CMB(PtI)	Charing Cross Hospital, London
Warner	H.J.		Imperial Cancer Research Fund, London
Warren	Mrs. J.	SRN, HV	Coventry AHA
Waters	Miss E.R.	SRN, SCM	Nottinghamshire AHA(T)
Watkins	Dr. M.E.	MB,BS,MRCS,LRCP,MSCM	Enfield and Harringay AHA
Watkins	* Mrs. P.	SRN, SCM, BTA, DN	Buckinghamshire AHA
Watkins	* Dr. R.P.	MB, ChB, DRCOG	Aylesbury, Buckinghamshire
Watkins	Miss T.M.	SRN	North Middlesex Hospital, London
Watson	Miss M.	SRN	Meyerstein Institute of Radiotherapy, London
Watts	Mrs. P.E.	SEN	Wessex Radiotherapy Centre
Waugh	Miss J.A.	SRN, SCM, HV, QN	Greenwich HD
Weatherby	Mrs. J.	RSCN, SRN	General Hospital, Plymouth
Webster	Miss I.	Nursing Officer	Royal Marsden Hospital, Surrey
Weir	Miss J.	RSCN, SRN, CMB(PtI)	General Hospital,Newcastle-upon-Tyne
Wenban	Miss E.	Social Worker	West Sussex Social Services
Westgate	Mrs. B.		S.-W. Thames Regional Cancer Council
Whatley	Miss N.I.	SRN, SCM, HV, DN	Gwent AHA
Wheatley	Mrs. M.E.	SRN, CMB(PtI),HV	Kingston and Richmond AHA
Whelan	Miss J.M.	RGN	Lothian Health Board, Scotland
Wheldon	Mrs. M.A.	BTA Cert.	Leicester
Whitehouse	K.W.	Staff Nurse	Royal Hospital, Wolverton
Whittaker	Mrs. S.	BSc.	University of Manchester
Whur	Dr. P.	BVMS,PhD,DVM,MRCVS	Research Department, MCMF
Wigfield	Dr. W.J.	MA,MB,BChir,DPH,MFCM	East Sussex AHA
Wilkinson	* Miss E.F.	SRN, SCM, BTA, HV	Hertfordshire AHA

Surname	Name	Qualifications	Affiliation
Willard	Mrs. D.K.	SRN, SCM, DN	Bath HD
Williams	Mrs. A.	SRN	West Middlesex Hospital
Williams	Dr. B.T.	MD, DPH, DPM, MFCM	Trent RHA
Williams	* Dr. D.C.	BSc., PhD, FRIC	Research Department, MCMF
Williams	Dr. D.T.	MB, BS	Chiddingfold, Surrey
Williams	Mrs. E.M.	MIHE	Tenovus Cancer Information Centre
Williams	Com. H.W.	OBE, FRCS	Salvation Army, London
Williams	Miss I.	SRN, SCM	Wirral AHA
Williams	Mrs. K.	SRN, SCM	Clwyd North HD
Williams	Miss M.F.	SRN, RSCN, SCM, ON	Worcester HD
Williams	* * Miss O.	SRN, SCM, DN	Surrey AHA
Williams	* * Mrs. P.	SRN, ONC	Holme Tower Nursing Home, MCMF
Willows	Mrs. M.M.	SRN, SCM, RFN	Charing Cross Hospital, London
Wilson	Miss J.H.	SRN	Salford AHA(T)
Wilson	Mrs. S.	Social Worker	Leicestershire County Council
Wilson	Mrs. Y.F.	SRN	Cleveland AHA
Wingfield	Miss J.A.		Royal Free Hospital, London
Withnall	Miss S.R.	BSc.	Medical Research Council, London
Withnell	Dr. A.	MD, FFCM, DPH	Gloucestershire AHA
Wood	Miss E.	SRN, FSRT	North Nottingham HD
Wood	Mrs. J.M.	SRN, DN, PWT	Lewisham, Lambeth & Southwark AHA(T)
Wood	M.A.	MIHE, AIPR	Ulster Cancer Foundation
Wood	M.E.	HND	Research Department, MCMF
Woodhouse	Miss J.		Salvation Army, London
Woodward	Mrs. M.A.	SRN, QN	Greenwich HD
Worsfold	Miss I.	SRN, SCM, HV	Cambridgeshire AHA(T)
Wray	Miss M.	SRN, SCM, HV, DN	London
Wright	Mrs. E.J.	SRN	Hertfordshire AHA
Wright	Miss S.J.	SRN	Grove Park Hospital, London

Young	Mrs. E.M.	SRN,SCM,BTA,DN,PWI	Hertfordshire County Council
Young	Dr. J.A.	MB, BCh, BAO, BA	Royal Infirmary, Glasgow
Young	* Miss K.G.	SRN, RSCN	Benenden Chest Hospital, Kent
Ziervogel	Miss C.	Social Worker	St. Thomas's Hospital, London
Zino	Dr. F.J.	MB, BS, MRCS, LRCP	British Broadcasting Corp., London

* Delegates attending both symposia.

ABBREVIATIONS

D.H.S.S.	Department of Health and Social Security
M.C.M.F.	Marie Curie Memorial Foundation
R.H.A.	Regional Health Authority
A.H.A.(T)	Area Health Authority (Teaching)
A.H.A.	Area Health Authority
H.D.	Health District

REPRESENTATIVES FROM THE MEDIA

British Broadcasting Corporation
        Finnish Overseas Service
        World Service
        Radio Science Unit
        Science and Features Department
        Science Correspondent
        Television News
Community Care
Daily Telegraph
Evening Standard
General Practitioner
Health and Social Service Journal
Hospital Life
Mims Magazine
Modern Medicine
Nursing Mirror
Nursing Times
Nursing Week
Physiotherapy
Press Association
Update Review
World Medicine
Lady Dawe, Free Lance
Mrs. Wendy Robinson, Free Lance

M.C.M.F. STAFF

Barleycorn	Miss F.G.	Welfare Department
Laxman	Miss K.	Secretariat
Lister	Mrs. S.	Secretariat
Looker	Miss L.	Secretariat
Raw	Mrs. V.	Secretariat
Reid	M.	Welfare Department
Steward	G.D.	Homes and Welfare Officer
Sturgess	P.A.	Assistant Secretary,MCMF.
Thistle	Miss V.	Secretariat